T0342271

Luminos is the Open Access monograph publishing program
from UC Press. Luminos provides a framework for preserving and
reinvigorating monograph publishing for the future and increases
the reach and visibility of important scholarly work. Titles published
in the UC Press Luminos model are published with the same high
standards for selection, peer review, production, and marketing as
those in our traditional program. www.luminosoa.org

A

Philip E. Lilienthal

B O O K

The Philip E. Lilienthal imprint
honors special books
in commemoration of a man whose work
at University of California Press from 1954 to 1979
was marked by dedication to young authors
and to high standards in the field of Asian Studies.
Friends, family, authors, and foundations have together
endowed the Lilienthal Fund, which enables UC Press
to publish under this imprint selected books
in a way that reflects the taste and judgment
of a great and beloved editor.

The publisher and the University of California Press Foundation
gratefully acknowledge the generous support of the
Philip E. Lilienthal Imprint in Asian Studies, established
by a major gift from Sally Lilienthal.

A Life of Worry

ETHNOGRAPHIC STUDIES IN SUBJECTIVITY

Tanya Luhrmann, Editor

A Life of Worry

Politics, Mental Health, and Vietnam's Age of Anxiety

———

Allen L. Tran

UNIVERSITY OF CALIFORNIA PRESS

University of California Press
Oakland, California

Suggested citation: Tran, A. L. *A Life of Worry: Politics, Mental Health, and Vietnam's Age of Anxiety*. Oakland: University of California Press, 2023.
DOI: https://doi.org/10.1525/luminos.162

All interior photos by author.

Library of Congress Cataloging-in-Publication Data

Names: Tran, Allen L., author.
Title: A life of worry : politics, mental health, and Vietnam's age of anxiety /
    Allen L. Tran. Other titles: Ethnographic studies in subjectivity ; 17.
Description: Oakland, California : University of California Press, [2023] |
    Series: Ethnographic studies in subjectivity ; 17 | Includes bibliographical
    references and index.
Identifiers: LCCN 2023003597 (print) | LCCN 2023003598 (ebook) |
    ISBN 9780520392168 (paperback) | ISBN 9780520392175 (ebook)
Subjects: LCSH: Anxiety—Social aspects—Vietnam. | Anxiety—
    Political aspects—Vietnam. | Mental health—Social aspects—Vietnam.
Classification: LCC BF575.A6 T736 2023 (print) | LCC BF575.A6 (ebook) |
    DDC 152.4/609597—dc23/eng/20230501

LC record available at https://lccn.loc.gov/2023003597
LC ebook record available at https://lccn.loc.gov/2023003598

32 31 30 29 28 27 26 25 24 23
10 9 8 7 6 5 4 3 2 1

CONTENTS

ILLUSTRATIONS

FIGURES

ACKNOWLEDGMENTS

I like to read a book's acknowledgments first to get the story behind the stories. In my favorite stories about Vietnam that I heard as a child, the country was a place of an idyllic beauty that could easily slide into something dangerous. The beaches in Vũng Tàu, where my mother grew up, have a deceptively strong undertow. Guava branches in Sơn Tây made the best slingshots for my father and his friends to shoot at birds and each other with. The stakes in the stories from my parents' last years in the country before they moved to the United States in 1975 became starker yet more ambiguous. Risk, desperation, and cruelty yielded to somehow even more gutting acts of compassion and honor. So I suppose my first thanks should go to my parents and my aunts and uncles for the stories that sparked my interest in Vietnam and the sacrifices they made that allowed that curiosity to become a vocation. Listening to these stories with me were my brother and our twenty-two cousins. Thank you for the nonstop mischief, inside jokes, drama, and commiseration, as well as the stories of your own.

My deepest gratitude, however, goes to the people in Ho Chi Minh City whose generosity and patience I will never be able to repay. My colleagues at the Southern Institute for Social Sciences patiently explained to me the contours of sentiment (*tình cảm*) and demonstrated it to me every time I saw them. Prof. Văn Thị Ngọc Lan, Bùi Linh Cường, Nguyễn Đặng Minh Thảo, Hà Thúc Dũng, and especially Lê Thế Vững and Nguyễn Cúc Trâm went above and beyond to support my research. The psychiatrists and psychotherapists I spoke with are laying the foundations for future generations of mental health care workers, yet they made time in their busy schedules to share their approach to treating anxiety, demonstrating their conviction and determination in the process. Their patients and clients were often even more giving of their time and energy under difficult circumstances. Most of all, I want to acknowledge the people I call Hoa, Hải, and especially Trâm for trusting me with their stories. Their lives have unfolded over the past decade in ways I certainly did not see coming. In particular, the twists and turns in Hải's life after the events described in chapter 6 warrant another book. But all three of them faced trials, successes, and the long, discouraging stretches of stagnation in between with their sense of humor intact, and they continue to seek out new ways of thinking about their world.

I first learned to think about the world like an anthropologist as an undergraduate at the University of California, Los Angeles, where classes taught by Doug Hollan, Jason Throop, and Linda Garro sent me on my way. This project took shape under the guidance of Tom Csordas, my primary advisor, and Janis Jenkins, first at Case Western Reserve University and then at the University of California, San Diego (UCSD). Whenever I got lost in the weeds of social theory, Tom's ability to pinpoint where I took a wrong turn always left me shaking my head in disbelief—*how did he do that?*—when I left his office. In terms of my research topic, I have long followed the trail set by Janis's detailed and empathic work on how mental health and illness are experienced at the level of the individual and the collective. At UCSD, Steve Parish became and still is my role model of the anthropologist as writer, and Suzanne Brenner, Eddy Malesky, and Yen Le Espiritu gave much-needed counsel on the politics and logistics of conducting research in Southeast Asia. Just as important as my committee to my progression through graduate school were my fellow students, including Nicole Barger, Jon Bialecki, Waqas Butt, Esin Duzel, Ted Gideonse, Candler Hallman, Eric Hoenes, Nofit Itzhak, Tim Karis, Corinna Most, Jess Novak, Tim Shea, and Brendan Thornton. Eli Elinoff, Whitney Duncan, and Heather Spector Hallman deserve highlighted recognition for their support and motivation, then and now.

My colleagues in the department of sociology and anthropology at Bucknell University have given me more mentoring, and more of a sense of community, than I ever expected. I am grateful for Deb Abowitz, Karen Altendorf, Danny Alvord, Matt Baltz, Dannah Dennis, Elizabeth Durden, Sarah Egan, Lauren Fordyce, Natalie Kuhns, Stevie Rea, and Clare Sammells. Conversations with Deb Baney, Michelle Johnson, and Ned Searles carried me across the finish line more often than they know. Outside of my department, drinks, dinner clubs, and pub trivia with JiaJia Dong, Scott England, Qing Jiang, Leo Landrey, Alicia Hayashi Lazzarini, Heather Mechler, Christine Ngô, John Penniman, David Rojas, Sezi Seskir, Dan Temkin, and Bryan Vandevender have also been essential. Anna Baker and I cotaught an interdisciplinary class on anxiety, and her clinical expertise moved chapter 5 away from simple critique. My anxious Gen Z students' honesty about their own experiences and curiosity about others' always gave me more to think through. Chapter 7 was written with them in mind. Jonathan Bean, Erica

Delsandro, Annetta Grant, and Aaron and Marissa Mitchel made a small college town in Pennsylvania feel more like a home. Any place with my dog Roger seems like home, so thank you to Hadar Sayfan for opening hers in New York City to us.

Portions of this book have been presented at conferences for the American Anthropological Association, Association for Asian Studies, and Society for Psychological Anthropology and benefited from the engagement of panel organizers and discussants, including Amy Borovoy, Paul Brodwin, Tom Csordas, Byron Good, Hsuan-Ying Huang, Janis Jenkins, Ann Marie Leshkowich, Rebecca Lester, Andrea Muehlebach, Eugene Raikhel, Christina Schwenkel, Jason Throop, Ben Tran, Anita von Poser, Julia Vorhölter, Jie Yang, and Jarrett Zigon, among many others. Side conversations with Nick Bartlett, Elizabeth Carpenter-Song, Vivian Choi, Michael D'Arcy, Jenna Grant, Chris Kortright, Martha Lincoln, Abby Mack, Raphaëlle Rabanes, Sarah Rubin, and Michelle Stewart have become the highlight of these events. Merav Shohet has carefully read and reread almost everything I have written, an expression of her own excellent work on care and sacrifice. I look forward to all of us gathering together again, hopefully soon. My gratitude also goes to the audiences and participants at UCSD's Seminar in Psychological and Medical Anthropology and Science Studies Program; UCLA's Mind, Medicine, and Culture Seminar; Bucknell's Medical Humanities Working Group and Center for the Study of Race, Ethnicity, and Gender; the Framing (Dis)Orders Workshop at Washington University in St. Louis; and the Affective Arrangements in Therapeutic Settings Symposium at Freie Universität Berlin.

Ho Chi Minh City draws a brilliant and supportive network of scholars whose work grounds my own and always generates new ideas and connections to explore. Ethnographic research is exciting and fulfilling but can be so draining! Being able to vent or puzzle over something with fellow researchers is a gift, especially when done over a bowl of noodles and a crisp lager with ice or a bougie cocktail. *Dzô* to Erik Harms, Ann Marie Leshkowich, Hy Van Luong, and Christina Schwenkel for the insights into Vietnam studies; Ivan Small and Jamie Gillen for the laughs; Mitch Aso and Caroline Herbelin for the stickers and gifs; Alex Cannon, Hyunok Lee, Khải Thư Nguyễn, and Maria Stalford for the deep conversations and support; Claire Edington and Haydon Cherry for the gossip; and Sarah Grant for all of the above. Numerous research trips to Ho Chi Minh City were made possible by the National Science Foundation; UCSD's International, Comparative, and Area Studies Research Fund; and Bucknell's Scholarly Development Grant, International Research Travel Grant, and Tom Greaves Fund for Research or Curricular Development.

At UC Press, Kate Marshall and Chad Attenborough ushered this book through the publication process with more patience than I deserved. Thank you to Tanya Luhrmann for making the introduction to Kate. The generous and astute comments of three reviewers, one of whom was later revealed to be Nick Bartlett, sharpened my arguments and expanded their scope. Portions of chapters 3, 4, and 6 were previously published in *American Anthropologist*, the *Journal of the Royal Anthropological Institute*, and *Medical Anthropology Quarterly*.

My father, Lưu Tran, passed away as I was considering whether to pursue a career in anthropology. Shortly before he died, he told me that he wasn't worried about me. My mother, Julie Tran, worries about me more than anyone ever has or ever will. This book falls somewhere between their ways of worrying and would not have been possible without either. My brother, Brian Tran, is the storyteller of the family, and his book will be much better than mine. I am still trying to worry about/for him just enough. *Của bố mẹ, em.*

PART ONE

Forms of Anxiety

1

How to Worry

Bác Lan's kitchen did not have any windows. It was tucked in the back of the ground floor of her narrow four-story house in downtown Ho Chi Minh City, Vietnam, so the only light came from fluorescent tubes overhead and a television's blue-tinted glare that bounced off the room's cool, sterile surfaces: all tile, metal, glass, and plastic. Still, the room felt oddly comforting to me. Most Vietnamese kitchens are spotlessly utilitarian, with little decoration or personal ornamentation, but this one featured a breakfast nook framed underneath recessed walls and built-in shelves. On the shelves were figurines of Phúc Lộc Thọ (the trio of East Asian deities associated with prosperity, status, and longevity) and various Disney characters as well as framed photographs of Bác Lan, her husband Vũ, and their daughter "Mimi" (a family nickname). The biggest picture was of Bác Lan, smiling in front of a Cartier boutique in Paris during a trip to visit her sister. Of course, much of why I was drawn to this kitchen was due to Bác Lan herself, a cheerful fifty-nine-year-old who was always ready to receive unannounced visitors with mangos, lychees, dragonfruit, or whatever was in season. Because she was one of the few people in Ho Chi Minh City I knew who was actually born and raised there, I occasionally stopped by her home to ask her how the house, neighborhood, and city had changed.

Born into a wealthy family in what was then French colonial Saigon, Bác Lan grew up in the house with the windowless kitchen, but its layout was much different then. Commissioned by her grandfather, the house was built on a spacious plot on a wide, bustling boulevard. Even against the backdrop of the Second Indochina War—more commonly known outside of Vietnam as the "Vietnam War" but what most Vietnamese call the "American War"—Bác Lan had, by her account, a happy childhood spent playing with numerous cousins and schoolmates. Indeed, many native Saigonese recall the war as a time when the American presence brought an influx of capital into the city and describe it as a happy (*sung sướng*)[1] one. This characterization of the war era is no doubt a reaction to the one that followed, which many people, including Bác Lan, said was the most difficult period of their life. After the war ended in 1975, the state sought to improve all aspects of life in a newly reunified Vietnam through socialist transformation. However, Ho Chi Minh City residents' recollection of the following ten years emphasize the suffering (đau khổ) endured as a result of an oftentimes punitive regime change, government mismanagement, domestic economic stagnation, and chronic shortages of essential goods. Poverty, hunger, and malnutrition—already rampant from thirty years of war—worsened somehow. Bác Lan's father had walls built to divide the house into three separate units and sold the flanking residences to sustain the family through the transition of a newly reunified Vietnam.

"Nghịch lý," Vũ chimed in. A paradox! Himself a rumored supporter of the new regime, he went on to say that everything that the Saigonese had known until then was suddenly turned upside down. Streets once bustling with social and commercial activity became eerily calm. The poor were rewarded for their status as the proletariat, while Saigon's elite were punished as bourgeoisie sympathizers. The youthful Communist vanguard became more powerful than their elders, now vilified as feudal and superstitious. Parents were afraid of their children, not the other way around. Profound economic scarcity led to suspicion and distrust where there had once been generosity and fellowship. Many of the people I spoke with during my research insisted to me that because of the war and its aftermath the Vietnamese had known more suffering than anyone else on the planet. Furthermore, Bác Lan and Vũ insisted that the Saigonese—or at least those who profited from an inflated wartime economy—suffered the most during that time because they had the steepest decline in quality of life. Everyone else in the country was used to hardship. For Bác Lan, the worst part was simply not knowing what would happen each day. Such uncertainty makes adequate planning for the future an impossibility, yet her every waking moment was still spent figuring out how to survive.

In 1986, a series of neoliberal reforms known as đổi mới (renovation) began to be gradually rolled out; by the early 1990s, signs of the country's economic revitalization were obvious. This process entailed the "normalization" (bình thường hoá) of Vietnam's relations with its former adversary the United States, but Bác Lan usually used the word bình thường lại, or "renormalize," to describe the era and the city's return to form. By now the owner of the house, Bác Lan rented out her front room to a photocopier repair shop, earning enough income for her and Vũ to retire comfortably and send Mimi to university. (It was around this time that she remodeled her kitchen.) With more and more storefronts and restaurants opening across the city, the street outside her house became busy "just like before," except that all the bicycles were replaced with motorbikes. Surely this was evidence, not only that life had become normal again, but that significant progress was happening.

Some nights, though, in the last moments before Bác Lan drifted to sleep, she would be dropped wide awake in a familiar feeling. It is some time between 1981 and 1985, and she is thinking about what to do next.

I discovered late into my initial fieldwork that Bác Lan's kitchen was designed by an American-trained architect. No wonder I felt at home there. Yet this unconscious reminder of home when I was far from it was unnerving. A few years later, the kitchen was torn down along with the walls that divided the ground floors of the three residences, reunited as a gleaming white car dealership.

HOW TO WORRY

Bác Lan is hardly alone in her worries. Insecurity of all stripes makes headlines around the world. For example, economic volatility in a globalized marketplace now has worldwide effects. As precarity becomes the rule rather than the exception, once stable political orders buckle under austerity measures and the rise of antiestablishment political movements, giving lie to the idea that they were even stable to begin with. We have yet to see the worst of global climate change, but we know it is coming and perhaps has already begun. The fact that most of us cannot fathom what "it" will look like makes the associated uncertainty that much more disquieting. Of course, these persistent problems have been exacerbated by the COVID-19 pandemic, the effects of which on our physical and mental health are persistent yet still unclear. Anxiety and stress disorders are the most common types of mental illness in the world and are the sixth leading cause of disability (Baxter et al. 2014b). At any given moment, one in fourteen people on the planet suffer from an anxiety disorder (Baxter et al. 2013). In the United States, that figure is one in four (WHO World Mental Health Survey Consortium 2004), representing a twentyfold increase since the *Diagnostic and Statistical Manual of Mental Disorders, Third Edition (DSM-III)* standardized the diagnosis of anxiety disorders almost fifty years ago.[2] It should be little surprise that anxiety is trending on and off social media platforms. The number of people who Googled anxiety has doubled in less than a decade, and the hashtag #ThisIsWhatAnxietyFeelsLike has millions of posts on Twitter (Williams 2017). Social media campaigns by various mental health collectives, such as the National Alliance on Mental Illness, advocate that "it's OK to not be OK" in an attempt to destigmatize discussion of one's mental health problems. Being OK with not being OK has become not just a mantra of the times but a structure of feeling as well (Williams 1977).

Anxiety is the general apprehension of threats to what we hold as essential to our being and its flourishing. As an anthropologist, I focus on its relational dimensions. Indeed, anxiety can itself be considered a kind of relationship between the self and a world of uncertainty. An unfortunate turn of events may provoke a wide range of emotional reactions, but what distinguishes anxiety from those other feelings is that it revolves around what might happen, not just an existing danger. It is a register of lived experience that invokes questions of meaning and deadlines, headaches and being-in-the-world; these questions are usually "what if?" questions. Anxiety ranges and cycles from the catastrophic to moments of indecision and a "sense of dull disquiet" (O'Gorman 2015, 25). Circumstances that have not yet come to pass and exist because we imagine them as a possibility may be more pressing—even more real—than what is already over and done with. Worse yet, at times we do not know what we are afraid of, and this suggests that what is so troubling about anxiety is rooted not in a particular object of fear but in something about ourselves and our ability to respond to the unknown. Anxieties are a part of us yet lie beyond our ability to know, let alone control, them. "What is there so fearful as the expectation of evil tidings delayed?" the nineteenth-century writer Mary Wollstonecraft Shelley wrote. "For then the heart no longer sickens with disappointed hope." The answer to her question may be found in her most famous work, *Frankenstein* (1818), with its themes of alienation, ambition, and the unanticipated consequences of scientific progress.

Based on ethnographic research conducted during the periods 2007–09, 2015–16, and 2019–20, with several summers of fieldwork in between, *A Life of Worry* is a cultural biography of the anxieties that take on a life of their own in Ho Chi Minh City.[3] Biographies of noted individuals suggest formative narratives of identity. As a genre, they typically frame their subject as an autonomous protagonist to speak truth to power. However, as I loosely conceive it, the cultural biography is neither a hero's journey nor a cautionary tale. Applying a biographical lens to anxiety, stress, and worry focuses less on the individuals who experience them—though certainly those individuals populate the study that follows. It places anxiety just outside of the context of an individual's psyche to examine its own agentive force and how it is sustained by social relationships and institutions. Following Fassin and Rechtman's (2009) analysis of trauma's hold on the medical, legal, and public imagination, this book traces the epistemologies and discourses of new scientific paradigms and a shifting moral economy. But I also explore how worries can take on a life of their own as they travel in and out of the clinic as well as between individuals. People often know that they worry needlessly and return to those worries compulsively, unable to either avoid future suffering or stop themselves from the torment of anxiety. These feelings do more than embellish moments in people's lives. They have far-reaching social repercussions that move across social relationships and institutions. Anxiety can define the subject but can also exceed it.

This book offers a conceptual approach to anxiety that is different from how we are often trained to think about it. The dominant perspectives from philosophy, psychology, and, increasingly, neuroscience frame anxiety as an emotional state, a pathological symptom, a biochemical process, or an existential condition. By individualizing and universalizing the experience of anxiety, these conceptualizations obscure the critical role of anxiety's social context. Thus, I conceptualize anxiety as a practice—something we do and perform in addition to feel and experience—that creates and sustains social relationships. And as with all social practices, anxiety is not entirely innate. The process of worry entails caring about an object and imagining a future that threatens that object, actions that are profoundly shaped by social and political forces. Put simply, we learn how to worry. Thus, I examine the cultural and personal patterning of mundane and extraordinary, as well as normative and pathological, forms of anxiety and how local systems of knowledge, relationships, and practices inform and are informed by anxiety. If we pay attention to how people in Vietnam confide their own specific anxieties to their families, friends, colleagues, doctors, counselors, and the occasional anthropologist, we can also glean their attempts to articulate new ways of living in a rapidly changing society. Going beyond what people say about their worries to the social and institutional construction of anxiety requires attending to multiple levels of analysis and the resonances between them. As a phenomenological study of anxiety and global capitalism in Ho Chi Minh City, this book analyzes that feeling akin to when you trip and "the ground is rushing up at you before you land" (Solomon 2001) and situates it in the broader context of the ground that shifted beneath your feet in the first place. If emotions are interpretations of problems, then examining the state construction of affect reveals how the historical, ideological, and embodied registers of those problems connect each other (Jenkins 1991; Ngai 2007).

Despite their global prevalence, anxiety and anxiety disorders have received sporadic anthropological attention.[4] This is all the more striking given the extensive literature within medical anthropology on other forms of mental health concerns stemming from the dangers of social experience (Kleinman et al. 1997). These studies examine the continuum between normal and pathological forms of emotional experience and the medical and political process of setting a boundary between them. While people with depression (Kitanaka 2011), trauma (Daniel 1996; Jenkins and Cofresi 1998; Lester 2013), and substance abuse (Garcia 2010; Bartlett 2020) often focus on coming to terms with the past, anxiety is primarily oriented toward the future. The unknowability of what lies ahead is not anxiety's only source of ambiguity. In today's transnational capitalism, the nature of the sociopolitical itself cultivates more ambient feelings that are perhaps less forceful than the political passions of fear and anger but no less effective (Virno 2004; Ngai 2007). Anxiety draws our attention to the precarity of everyday experiences and how it is linked to relations of gendered care, classed aspirations, and moral selfhood.

A Life of Worry opens in Bác Lan's kitchen because anxiety does not need the darkest recesses of the soul to take root, though a dimly lit room does not hurt. After all, Bác Lan is not a particularly nervous person. Yet the potential for anxiety surrounds her. The states of her mind, house, and hometown intersect to blur the boundaries between past and present, as well as between self and other.

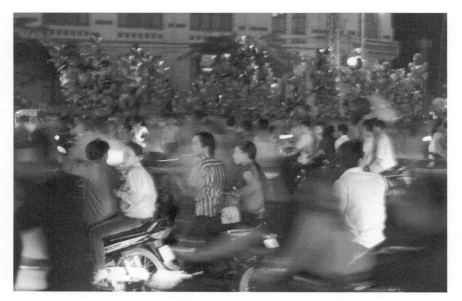

FIGURE 1. A popular way to unwind in the early 2000s, *di chơi* (to go play) entails cruising through the city on motorbikes with friends.

These convergences, which register alternately as dissociation or signs of economic progress, may appear to be unrelated, but anxiety can arise from seemingly innocuous and chance circumstances. It is not the sole product of individual-level factors because it does not reside within individuals. Rather, much like selfhood, anxiety exists somewhere between individuals and the world, demonstrating that the self does not exist independently of its relation to the world. In anxiety, people find themselves "thrown" from the familiar, suddenly not at home in the world (Heidegger 1962). Though Bác Lan is thrown back to the 1980s for only a second, the effect lingers. The paradox of the postwar lean years that Vũ describes and the post-reform return to "normal" question what all that suffering was for. This question starkly contrasts with the official narrative of personal sacrifices made for the benefit of a Communist victory (Shohet 2013). Furthermore, the return of something—whether it is the postwar lean years (if just for a moment), the ground floor of a house, or a capitalist economy—is uncanny because it brings the familiar to an unfamiliar context (Freud 1919). Although Bác Lan and her contemporaries are still trying to determine the meaning of Vietnam's traumatic history, it is important for us to avoid explaining away the confusion of anxiety. Liberal discourses of the emotions privilege them as the site of intimate self-knowledge, but anxiety alienates us from the world to reveal the self faced with its own indeterminacy.

Saigon and Ho Chi Minh City

A woman on the cusp of a promising career comes under increasing pressure from her parents to abandon it in order to marry and have children. A market vendor struggles to find the money to pay her child's tuition. A student crams for finals; his classmate is concerned that he has not felt the urge to study all semester. A patient at the Ho Chi Minh City Psychiatric Hospital who has just been diagnosed with depression wonders how she will pay for her medication, how she will manage her work and family obligations with an illness, and whether or not she will one day "go crazy" (*bị điên*). That the set of concerns that preoccupy Ho Chi Minh City residents—financial woes, work pressures, and family tensions—may seem so familiar or exceedingly ordinary to many of us is, in and of itself, remarkable given the tumult of Vietnam's recent history. For most people outside of the country, "Vietnam" has become synonymous with the "Vietnam War," oversimplifying both the country's past and its present. Although this book does not focus on that war, understanding its themes requires proper contextualization of the war and its legacy. Here, I briefly set the historical context of Ho Chi Minh City before I delve into the effects of specific policies in the following sections.

Then an outpost of the Khmer empire called Prey Nokor, Saigon came under jurisdiction of Vietnam in 1698 as part of its Southward March (Nam Tiến) from Hanoi during the fifteenth through eighteenth centuries. Near the fertile Mekong Delta, it quickly expanded under Vietnamese rule and developed a national reputation as a place of relative wealth, ease, and leisure that it maintains to this day. When the French colony of Indochina (encompassing present-day Vietnam, Cambodia, and eventually Laos) was established in 1887, Saigon was named its first capital and has since borne the strongest Western influence in the region. On September 2, 1945, the Communist revolutionary Hồ Chí Minh read the Proclamation of Independence to a crowd of thousands at Ba Đình Square in Hanoi to announce the founding of the Democratic Republic of Vietnam (DRV) and Vietnam's independence from France. The ensuing First Indochina War was fought between the Viet Minh (Việt Nam Độc Lập Đồng Minh, League for the Independence of Vietnam), led by Hồ Chí Minh, and French and pro–French Vietnamese forces. The Geneva Conventions of 1954 ended the war with the partitioning of Vietnam into the DRV in the North and the State of Vietnam, renamed the Republic of Vietnam (ROV) a year later, in the South. Over the next year, nearly one million political refugees, known as the '54 Northerners (*Bắc 54*), relocated from the North to the South.

The Second Indochina War set the DRV, the southern-based National Liberation Front with their military wing the Viet Cong (Việt Nam Cộng Sản, Vietnamese Communists), and Communist supporters, including the Soviet Union and China, against the ROV and the United States with additional support from South Korea, Australia, and other anticommunist allies. During the twenty years of this undeclared war, over three million Vietnamese combatants and civilians were killed, and tens of thousands more died after the war due to unexploded ordnance or the chemical defoliant known as Agent Orange. Moreover, millions in Cambodia and Laos were killed during and after the war. Vietnam was "reunified" when North Vietnam took Saigon, the southern capital, on April 30, 1975, and thereby ended one of the twentieth century's most controversial and devastating wars. However, as Viet Thanh Nguyen (2016, 4) writes, "all wars are fought twice, the first time on the battlefield, the second time in memory." A year later, Saigon was officially renamed Ho Chi Minh City, but most people in the country still refer to it informally as Saigon.

For many in Ho Chi Minh City, the immediate postwar period was worse than the conflict. What is described in state discourse as the liberation (*giải phóng*) of South Vietnam from foreign occupation was interpreted by many southerners as its defeat. This period was hardly a time of peace, as Vietnam invaded and eventually occupied Cambodia in 1978 (i.e., the Third Indochina War) and fought a brief but intense border conflict with China in 1979. Meanwhile, attempts to reconstruct the war-torn landscape, infrastructure, and economy were hampered by punitive international policies and trade embargoes designed to isolate the newly formed Socialist Republic of Vietnam. Many Ho Chi Minh City residents found that the biggest threats, however, came not from forces outside of the country but from within. The new regime sent some three hundred thousand ROV supporters, including soldiers and civil servants, to reeducation camps (*trại học tập cải tạo*), where sentences often lasted three to ten years. Devised to develop the hinterlands, collectivist farms in New Economic Zones were staffed with representatives of the old order (such as capitalists and Catholic priests), social undesirables (such as drug addicts and commercial sex workers), and urbanites who were displaced by the one million '75 Northerners (*Bắc 75*) who took high-ranking positions in the South soon after reunification.

Already implemented gradually in the (more collectively oriented) North, command-economy socialism was abruptly imposed on the South. The cosmopolitan modernity that Saigon evoked as the "Paris of the Orient" vanished overnight under a northern ethos of austerity. For the South's urban elite, a socialist future was "a regression to a premodern state bereft of the civilizing influence of middle-class education, manners, and respectability" (Leshkowich 2014a, 14). The new regime replaced private enterprise with a much-hated system of subsidies and vouchers that came to symbolize the failures and horrors of state-mandated collectivism. In the process, the much-vaunted entrepreneurial spirit of the Saigonese became delegitimized. With no more legal marketplaces or storefronts, long queues formed for basic necessities that were rationed out by the government. Waiting half a day for cooking oil, with no assurances there would be any left by the time one got to the head of the line, left people unsure whether to laugh or cry (*dở khóc dở cười*; MacLean 2008). This system was so poorly managed that poverty, famine, and material scarcity became widespread. Already on the brink from three decades of war, Vietnam's poverty worsened as a result of mismanagement, natural disasters, and punitive international sanctions. Hundreds of thousands of refugees fled political persecution and economic deprivation with the hope of resettling permanently in the West. These attempts to escape, often on small boats built only for short fishing expeditions, were themselves dangerous. Some estimate that for each person who arrived at a refugee camp in Hong Kong, Thailand, the Philippines, Indonesia, Malaysia, or Singapore, another died at sea (Osborne 1980).

However, fates changed in 1986 when neoliberal reforms known as *đổi mới* (renovation) introduced a "market economy with socialist orientations" (*kinh tế thị trường với hướng dẫn chủ nghĩa xã hội*), or market socialism. Thirty years of rapid economic growth—after a long civil war and a decade of socialist collectivization with disastrous results—has made Vietnam one of late capitalism's most celebrated success stories. For example, 70 percent of Vietnamese lived below the official poverty line at the end of the war in 1975. By 1992, when the early effects of *đổi mới* became broadly evident to Ho Chi Minh City residents, 58 percent were in poverty. Today, only 3 percent are (World Bank & Ministry of Planning and Investment of Vietnam 2016). (However, much of the poverty is concentrated in ethnic minority communities, a reflection of the persistent disparities throughout the country.) The general reduction in poverty had the World Bank reclassify Vietnam as a middle-income country in 2010, a remarkable achievement for a country that was, in living memory, one of the poorest in the world. These economic changes provide Ho Chi Minh City residents with opportunities to reimagine Vietnam's place in the global capitalist economy and envision its next steps toward global modernity (Hoang 2015). The national story that many Vietnamese tell themselves about themselves is one of optimism, development, and prosperity.

Nowhere is this narrative of national progress more salient than in the country's financial center of Ho Chi Minh City. With over thirteen million residents, the largest and most cosmopolitan city in the country was already primed to reenter the global economy and, for many, has come to symbolize Vietnam's bright future under neoliberal policies (Drummond 2000). The city that I arrived in to conduct my initial research from 2007 to 2009 was in perpetual motion. Almost every street I turned down was choked with construction crews and waves of motorbikes, and people in the midst of some urgent activity seemed to be everywhere. They sold cigarettes and rain ponchos from sidewalk carts and baguettes from bicycles, cracked bricks of ice to fit in glasses of sodas and coffee, wrapped *bánh mì* sandwiches in newspaper, and fanned the smoke of grilling pork into traffic. Storefronts for local boutiques and global chains, restaurants, and cafés were constantly opening, closing, and being replaced with something new to try. The return of capitalism to Ho Chi Minh City is bittersweet: sweet because it significantly raises living standards for everyone (even if some receive more of those benefits than others), bitter because it reminds people of what they had been missing during the subsidy era and all that could have been if the war had ended differently.[5] Indeed, *đổi mới* is haunted by the "uncanny specter of an alternative [and reascendant] South Vietnamese modernity preceding and perhaps succeeding socialism" (Small 2018, 21; Taylor 2001; Leshkowich 2014a).

The Subject of Anxiety

Yet all is not well in these boom times. Runaway inflation forces Ho Chi Minh City residents to work harder, with less to show for their efforts. Contending with urban decay, traffic congestion, and environmental pollutants on a daily and intimate basis further saps their physical and mental reserves. After *đổi mới* eased foreign media restrictions, allowing the publication of Western popular psychology pieces in newspapers, magazines, and self-help books, the concept of stress (*strés*) became trendy among urbanites. However, *strés* is not just a new label for familiar experiences. Rather, according to popular media accounts (Lam 2005), the Vietnamese are becoming "stressed" for the first time. But this is decidedly not the stress that comes with deprivation. Instead, now the province of the upwardly mobile, *strés* suggests the anxieties of overwhelming choice and multitasking. Thus, while *stress* may, ostensibly, refer to many difficult circumstances, in Vietnam its closest associations lie with the lifestyles of the purportedly modern middle class. Furthermore, rates of anxiety disorders throughout the country have risen steadily in recent years, with the National Association of Psychiatry warning that these figures likely underestimate the severity of a growing mental health crisis (Thuý Hạnh 2015). In recent years, Vietnamese youth have become increasingly open about their own struggles with everyday anxieties on social media platforms as they seek to destigmatize mental health problems. In a single generation, Ho Chi Minh City residents have gone from fearing war, famine, and poverty to worrying about sending children overseas to college, choosing the right cell phone, and maintaining their health into old age. Clearly, this represents an improvement in people's fates, but such profound changes, even ones for the better, can be difficult to adjust to. As much as people marvel at the speed of change under *đổi mới*, many struggle to understand it. Of course, uncertainties also accompanied the militaristic destruction and authoritarian rule of the past. Thus, the issue is not change itself but rather the particular quality of change of the post-reform era and, just as critically, how it alters the relationship between the self and the social.

What is distinct about anxiety's outlines in Ho Chi Minh City is how it has been transformed and redefined as an explicit problem in several domains of contemporary Vietnamese society. Many of the people I spoke with in Ho Chi Minh City reflected on the present by comparing it to the social and economic upheavals of the past. According to many of them, now that the country is modernizing so quickly, they have a greater amount of things to worry about than they did in the past. That is, the Vietnamese are more anxious now than ever before. To be sure, not all Ho Chi Minh City residents agreed with this statement, but enough of them did to make me pay attention to this purported "age of anxiety." I am less interested in verifying the accuracy of this claim than in following the logic behind it. What accounts for the simultaneous and seemingly paradoxical increase of economic prosperity, on one hand, and anxiety, worry, and stress on the other? How do people adapt to their new economic reality? Why does the country's transition to a market economy become understood through the lens of worry and embodied in an anxious register? Cultural commentators such as my interlocutors in Vietnam often seem to find themselves in a new age of anxiety because, after all, every historical moment is its own age of anxiety. Societies vary in their orientation to risk, fear, and anxiety, and different objects of concern may come to define a historical moment.[6] The phrase *age of anxiety* typically refers to the modern world and its perils. If, indeed, today's stakes are not as high as they used to be, they are at least more ambiguous. The notion that Vietnam's current historical moment is an age of anxiety reflects not so much a quantitative change in anxiety but instead its redefinition as it gets linked to new forms of insecurity.

What people fear and how they express and act upon that fear is, in some important way, constitutive of who they are, and Ho Chi Minh City's new worries take us across some of Vietnam's most critical social changes. How much worry one can or should endure is at the heart of ongoing debates over what constitutes a good life and a moral person in Ho Chi Minh City. I trace these debates across various settings to examine the diverse ways that people negotiate and transform their worries. Chief among these are the therapeutic contexts, such as psychiatric clinics and counseling centers, where the most intense struggles over the new meaning of worry take root. The psychological and medical sciences have become the primary wellspring of those technologies of the self that are used to adapt to emerging demands for the self. These means of imbuing anxiety with personal meaning and individual purpose both complement and contradict each other, but all of them are marshalled as evidence of the triumphs and failures of development.

The psychic and social foundations of anxiety in Vietnam have been laid by the history of the medical and psychological sciences, emerging forms of global capitalism, and new ways of setting the boundary between self and society. The process of self-discovery does not simply uncover an enduring and essential component of oneself but rather articulates it in publicly accessible forms. As people become subject to more sources and forms of anxiety, they must learn how to cope with them. However, in the process of learning how to worry in culturally specific ways, they also adopt new conventions of personhood. The subject of anxiety is the self oriented toward a future through technologies of the self designed to cope with insecurity and precarity. The rise of anxiety as a widespread social condition is the product of these new ways of relating to the self, others, and the world.

ANXIETIES ABOUT ANXIETIES

The paradoxes of Vietnam's age of anxiety make it clear that the severity of threats to a person's physical safety, self-esteem, or social status cannot adequately predict their level of anxiety. This suggests that anxiety is not merely a proportional outcome of potential stressors. Rather, it is the result of how people relate to an uncertain world. Thus, an ethnographic framework for anxiety should account for not just the level of danger or the fortitude of the self but also the way they interface with each other. Cross-cultural research on the emotions emphasizes their variation, construction, and regulation through cultural discourses, roles, and institutions (Lutz and Abu-Lughod 1990). More recently, scholars have called for greater attention to the sensory dimensions of affects that circulate throughout communities, as opposed to the language-bound study of the emotions (Seigworth and Gregg 2010).[7] Attending to how affective processes take form and, in turn, shape and exceed their surroundings is especially critical in the case of anxiety because it thrives in between established categories of experience. Thus, this book explores how selfhood is made and remade, how uncertainty is structured in a population, and how people interpret and respond to their anxieties. Here, drawing on some of the most influential theories of anxiety, I outline a conceptualization of anxiety in relation to a shifting cultural politics of the self. In the following sections, I will address the questions of the structure of uncertainty ("the age of anxiety" and "middle-class aspirations and moralities") and people's reactions to it ("the psy-turn").

We often imagine anxiety to be a universal problem—something that afflicts people no matter their historical or cultural context. However, an examination of the relatively recent history of the academic study of anxiety reveals a broad range of ways of grappling with it (May 1950). For example, anxiety was an intellectual problem for Enlightenment thinkers, a spiritual one for existentialists, and a libidinal and sexual one for psychoanalysts. Early twentieth-century physicians argued that excessive anxiety was a stress response to the rise of modern lifestyles and environments (Lutz 1991). The biochemical frameworks of the early twenty-first century, with their emphasis on nature over nurture, are evidence of an increasingly individualistic worldview (Horwitz 2013). Despite their many differences, philosophical, psychological, and medical approaches to anxiety have resulted in a diverse category of experience that, while awkward, nevertheless rings familiar to us. Does this familiarity, however, suggest universality, or is it the result of imposing our own ideas about anxiety onto the cultural particularities that most of these theories disregard? The extent to which anxiety is shared around the world depends on how it is defined. While some fear-based affective response to uncertainty is likely universal, the focus on anxiety's broadly shared features within the dominant paradigms has reproduced distinctly Western assumptions about emotion, selfhood, and risk. Indeed, much of how we understand anxiety is the product of both a prevailing state of scientific knowledge and particular configurations of self and society.

Initial theories of anxiety reflect their disciplinary origins in the tumult of the nineteenth century that gave rise to modernity in the West and its means of relating to the world, each other, and our selves. The emerging scientific, philosophical, and political ideals of the Enlightenment celebrated individual rights over communal-based obligations, and Cartesian dichotomies between the mind and the body led to a preoccupation with rational, mechanical phenomena. The technological advances of the Industrial Revolution yielded economic growth as well as new social formations as people moved away from established support systems and encountered new uncertainties. Indeed, the early twentieth-century social psychologist R. R. Willoughby famously described anxiety as "the most prominent characteristic of Occidental civilization." To this day, anxiety and modern lifestyles and identities retain a powerful association.

The earliest modern efforts to theorize anxiety, primarily within Euro-American philosophy and psychology, reacted against the rise of the technocratic, bureaucratic, and secular that turned virtually every aspect of life into something to calculate, compartmentalize, and control. Instead, they focused on the whole individual as a feeling and acting agent and highlighted the fundamentally emotional nature of human existence. For example, the philosopher Søren Kierkegaard (1884) called anxiety the "dizziness of freedom" because it results from an awareness that the ability to make one's own decisions creates different possibilities for oneself. Existential anxiety can happen to anyone as a normal event. It can even be morally valuable if one's response to it is personal growth and not retreat. For existentialists, anxiety is the key to deciphering the human condition yet also the central domain of male intellectuals (Ngai 2007). The broader question of who has access to the opportunities and resources needed to make their own decisions in order to achieve that growth is never addressed, however.

Conversely, Sigmund Freud (1936) focused on the pathological dimensions of anxiety as a foundational concept in psychoanalysis. For him, anxiety is the clinical manifestation of intrapsychic and unconscious conflicts and repressed demands. These so-called neurotic anxieties are not realistic assessments of one's own powerlessness or an outside threat but rather a flight from the libido's own demands.[8] Not all conflicts provoke neurotic anxiety. This is not to say that neurotic anxiety or repression may not be at play among the case studies in this book. Although I avoid applying wholesale the master discourse of psychoanalysis to my ethnographic data, I do attend to classically psychodynamic phenomena such as conflicting impulses that have no socially acceptable outlets. However, because this book is more concerned with anxiety's role in the intersubjective experience of social relationships than with the psychodynamic emphasis on the inner workings of the mind, I draw mainly from existentialism's close cousin phenomenology.

Philosophy's and psychology's intense focus on the nonconscious aspects of individual subjectivity overshadows the interpersonal dimensions of our emotional lives. To recover the significance of social processes in anxiety, we need an approach to selfhood that centers our capacity to form social relationships. Following Csordas (1994), I conceptualize selfhood as a process of orienting and becoming oriented to the world. Integral to this study is the insight that the self is not a "bounded, unique, more or less integrated motivational universe, a dynamic center of awareness, emotion, judgment, and action" (Geertz 1979, 229), as is commonly assumed in the West. Rather, it requires an Other, such as other people, material objects, or cultural values and ideologies, to orient toward in an ongoing process of becoming and possibility (Parish 2008). This framework for self-society relations is informed by phenomenological approaches to anthropology that complicate our understandings of the textures of subjective experience (Csordas 1990; Desjarlais 1992). Rather than taking people's lived experience at face value, these approaches interrogate how it unfolds and comes to be taken for granted (Csordas 1994). Focusing on how people engage with their social and physical environments as a contingent process sheds light on how experience may or may not achieve a meaningful and definite form through linguistic, symbolic, and embodied measures (Crapanzano 2004; Throop 2010). Emphasizing the coherent meanings that people ascribe to their experiences glosses over the ambiguities and ambivalences that are so characteristic of anxiety. From a phenomenological perspective, emotional states are much more than an adornment on an intrinsically rational agent. Rather, they reveal the fundamental ways people relate to the world, and perhaps none does so as sharply as anxiety (Heidegger 1962).

I argue that the development and experience of anxiety is inextricable from configurations of selfhood. Anxiety is unique among the emotions because it lacks an object (Barlow 2002). While people are happy to see a friend or jealous of someone else's good fortune, they are often unsure of why they feel anxious. Instead, they are only aware that they are afraid. If the self is produced and reproduced through engaging with an object, what happens in the absence of one? To answer this question, it is instructive to examine Kierkegaard's (1884) classic distinction between fear and anxiety. The difference between them is that between being acutely afraid of falling when you stand at a cliff's edge and experiencing the vague impulse to throw yourself off it. Because fear has a specific and immediate reason, attention becomes trained on the threatening object. People are able to reason a cogent explanation for their terror, orient themselves to the fear object, and mobilize for an appropriate fight-or-flight response. Their fright decreases when the object of fear is removed through concrete action.

Conversely, anxiety is the expectation of a threat when the danger is unknown. Jacques Lacan (2016) described anxiety as being trapped in a room with a three-meter-tall praying mantis while you are wearing a mask that you cannot see. How do you react to the giant insect when you do not know whether you look like its next meal or not? The absence of a fear object to orient toward makes the process of identifying and acting upon threats more fraught. Unsure of what one is afraid of, there is nothing to fight and nowhere to flee from as anxiety attacks from multiple directions. Because anxiety is a more generalized state of apprehension, the object is ignored in favor of the subjective condition (Freud 1952). Subsequently, it is felt as a cosmic experience that penetrates entire subjective universes. The diffuse apprehension and helplessness associated with it refers not only to its generalized physical sensations. After all, other emotions such as fear or anger are capable of saturating the body. Rather, anxiety's undifferentiated quality refers to an undermining of some foundational level of a person—their self-esteem or their experience of the self as a person (Bloch 1995). While fear can be mediated by establishing a security pattern to confront or avoid the object, in anxiety this security pattern may itself be under threat (Sullivan 1948). That is, not only is one compromised by a threat, but also the patterns of coping with it are under attack. People can neither objectify the threat nor separate themselves from it because the means to do so have been compromised by anxiety. Indeed, "the very perception with which we look will also be invited by anxiety" (May 1950, 191). Focused less on a threat than on the anticipated fragmentation of the self, anxiety faces the self with its own indeterminacy.

The notion that anxiety lacks an object runs counter to the way many people around the world have lately come to talk about their worries. For example, I have noticed in recent years that my own students and, increasingly, my colleagues refer to their "anxiety levels" as a way to gauge their mental health according to a metric. Contradicting Freud's (1952) claim that people have fears but are anxious, this reflects a growing vigilance over our emotional states and added pressure to conform to a new norm of mental health and wellness. Rather than dismiss this as an incorrect application of philosophical and psychoanalytic concepts, we should put popular notions and academic theories of anxiety in conversation with each other. The distinct objectless-ness of anxiety provides anthropologists with insights into the everyday making and unmaking of the self and prompts new questions about anxiety's role in social institutions. What kinds of social resources are used to channel unfocused fear into something more manageable, and to whom are they available? How can anxiety be converted into fear by identifying a threatening object? What gets left out in the process, and what happens if this process fails? How do cultural models of the self mediate anxiety? Is the fragmentation of selfhood experienced as an interruption or a continuation?[9] Moreover, the study of the intimate construction of selfhood need not be limited to the study of individual subjectivity. Indeed, a critical phenomenology that examines lived experience in relation to social and economic inequality has been used to shed light on immigration (Willen 2019), disasters and humanitarianism (Seale-Feldman 2020), and the war on drugs (Zigon 2019). Next, I examine how anxiety reflects the subjective experience of Vietnam's ongoing transition to a market economy. The freedom to imagine, choose, and navigate the possibilities of economic growth comes with a dizzying price.

THE AGE OF ANXIETY

Over a dinner of stir-fried beef and squash blossoms and a seafood hot pot, the Phạm siblings were trying to remember how their cousin had died. Yến, the fifty-five-year-old middle sister who was hosting us in her house, thought that he was picked off by a Cambodian sniper during the Third Indochina War in 1978. According to the oldest brother, Kiệt, sixty-eight, the cousin perished in a reeducation camp, an ordeal that Kiệt, a pilot in the ROV Air Force, had survived. The debate was never settled, however, because it led to more questions about the fates of other distant relatives or childhood friends and neighbors during the final days of the Second Indochina War and its chaotic aftermath. The answers to who had died, escaped, and were separated or reunited were told in spare but still gutting details. As Kiệt and his brothers and sisters raced to tell me story after story about the sacrifices made for and because of the nation's goal of mass collectivization, I could hear in the next room this family's next generation, most of whom were too young to remember much of the subsidy era. They were watching the latest American pop-culture phenomenon to make its way to Vietnam, the Disney Channel TV movie *High School Musical*. The film's message of being true to yourself celebrates individualism, but it ends with an upbeat song titled "We're All in This Together."

Six years later, in 2013, I visited Kiệt at his home—a platform raised halfway up from an apartment building's garage—and immediately noticed, but did not say, that he had become worrisomely gaunt. At one point, a young man with a shaggy beard climbed up the ladder and greeted me. "You don't recognize him, do you?" Kiệt said. It was his now twenty-two-year-old son Nam. I asked Nam what he had been doing since I last saw him with his cousins, but like many family elders in Vietnam, Kiệt took the liberty of answering the question for him. Nam had studied management at university and took additional Korean language classes, hoping to eventually find a job that would involve overseas travel. Upon graduating with high marks, Nam received job offers from several South Korean companies in Vietnam, but he wanted a career in a more creative field and so took a lucrative position as an events planner. Patting Nam's belly, Kiệt said the son had gotten fat while the father became thinner. Obviously proud of his son, Kiệt emphasized Nam's optimistic future. Nam would certainly rise from his family's poverty and maybe bring them out of it in the process. Conversely, Kiệt grew up in an affluent family and had hoped to become a lawyer one day. However, after reunification, his house and finances were seized by the new regime, and upon his release from the reeducation camp he worked as a barber (which is how I met him) because no formally recognized work was available for former ROV officers. Kiệt told me this in the same manner of detached bemusement with which he recounted his cousin's death. When I asked if this still upset him, he replied that initially he was furious but now the only thing he could do was to accept (*chịu*) his fate. At least Nam's generation, Kiệt said, can choose whatever they want to do.

The expansion of Nam's choices is largely credited to the *đổi mới* policies that, over the past three decades, have produced one of the fastest-growing economies in the world, second only to Vietnam's giant neighbor to the north, China. Indeed, neoliberalism, as both ideology and economic policy, promises freedom from constraints on growth and self-expression in the global marketplace, through individual freedom and choice (Harvey 2007). By the end of the 1980s, *đổi mới* had dismantled the unpopular rationing system of the subsidy period and established further engagement with the global economy and an "open door" (*mở cửa*) policy toward foreign direct investment (Beresford 2008). As in the former Soviet Bloc and across late-socialist Asia, private enterprise has since eclipsed the command economy as state-owned enterprises laid off most of their employees, once championed as the foundation of a socialist utopia (Yan 2010; Makovicky 2014). For example, under Maoism many Chinese were individuated by dismantling traditional kin and village organizations in order to foster allegiance toward the state (Greenhalgh and Winckler 2005). Furthermore, the implementation of neoliberal reforms disembedded people from state collectives used to define them in relation to the state (Yan 2010). Meanwhile, opportunities for work in Vietnam's informal sector became more plentiful as the United States lifted its trade embargo and normalized diplomatic relations in the 1990s. Marking the transition away from an agriculturally based economy, real estate development and construction, manufacturing, and more recently software development have brought significant amounts of speculation into the economy.

However, the Vietnamese Communist Party has deployed neoliberal principles in strategically uneven ways. For example, the decreased public presence of the state and increased volatility of the market have not come at the expense of socialist governance but rather reinforce state sovereignty (Nguyễn-Võ 2008). Thus, like so many other neoliberal projects throughout the region, the very incompleteness of *đổi mới* suggests that neoliberalism is best viewed not as a monolithic and autonomous entity but rather as a historically contingent set of divergent practices and institutions that stem from and encourage the deregulation of formerly public domains (Schwenkel and Leshkowich 2012). Given the irregular distribution of *đổi mới*, access to neoliberal ideals and practices varies by gender, class, generation, and regional background, resulting in fluid and hybridized political subjectivities (Pashigian 2012). Thus, rather than debating whether East and Southeast Asia can rightly be characterized as neoliberal or not, scholars should focus on how social and political actors navigate and adapt neoliberal principles for their own purposes.

The key to neoliberalism's mode of production may lie precisely in its ability to dominate through insecurity and precarity (Bourdieu 2003). Anticipation has become key to managing the risks of the *đổi mới* economy (Dao 2020). In a capitalist labor market, job requirements constantly change, and fears of being left behind prime people to reconfigure themselves according to market demands. As Marx observed of the origins of capitalism, people become alienated not only from others but also from themselves as a result of economic competition. That is, people's relationships to each other both reflect and become their attitudes toward themselves; alienation from others eventually becomes a form of self-alienation (May 1950). The affective milieu of contemporary global capitalism has become more diffuse and ambiguous than the political passions of fear and anger that characterize Hobbesian theories of modern sovereignty. Rather, the ambient flatness of the "sentiments of disenchantment" like anxiety, cynicism, and distraction have become integral to capitalist modes of production (Virno 2004).

To investigate the affective implications of neoliberal policies for self and personhood, anthropologists have turned to Michel Foucault's notion of the technologies of the self, or the tools people use to transform their own conduct, bodies, and minds so as to achieve "a certain state of happiness, purity, wisdom, perfection, or immortality" (Foucault 1988, 18). How people submit to neoliberal regimes and are themselves changed in the process is guided by a set of discourses that promotes a sense of reflexivity, most notably about the self, at all levels of society. Neoliberal reforms demand and rely on cultivating a new type of citizen who can cope with the withdrawal of the state from public life: someone who is flexible, autonomous, and oriented to an ethics of personal responsibility (Rose 1999; Brown 2003). "Neoliberal selfways" promote an ongoing project of self-entrepreneurialism, personal growth, and fulfillment as the basis for well-being, and a "freedom from constraint that affords an experience of radical abstraction from context" (Adams et al. 2019, 191). With social and personal identities now less fixed by long-standing norms, people become entrepreneurs of their own selves: objects to be manipulated to suit the demands of the capitalist marketplace (Giddens 1991). As both the seller and the commodity to be sold on the market, they are put into conflict over their own inner values of themselves and develop a sense of self-worth that depends on forces beyond their own control (Illouz 2007). Furthermore, not only do people learn new occupational skills to become upwardly mobile, but they must also apply these principles to their inner self; the accumulation of capital becomes not an end but a means of reinventing the self (Freeman 2014).

However, the Foucauldian emphasis on often abstract discourses yields a passive figure that seems wholly saturated by market principles. Here, people have virtually no choice but to become ideal neoliberal subjects. Focusing on the hybrid assemblages that result from encounters with demands for self-responsibility and autonomy works against a monolithically "neoliberal self" (Ong and Zhang 2008; Freeman 2014), and documenting the specificities of Vietnam's historical and cultural context in addition to *đổi mới*'s effects on personhood avoids overreaching with any claims of a "neoliberal self" (Leshkowich 2014b). Because purported neoliberal traits break considerably from the traits of collectivism that Vietnamese often use to describe themselves as a nation (see chapters 2 and 3), many people struggle with how to adopt them. Indeed, while Ho Chi Minh City residents engage with neoliberal discourses of the self, this process is neither straightforward nor inevitable. Close attention to ethnographic and historical detail reveals that qualities that may coincide with neoliberal imperatives are, in fact, supported by socialist and Confucian regimes of selfhood.

Ethnographic analyses of neoliberalism need not stop at documenting the cultural and historical differences in personhood that conflict and interfere with ideals related to self-determination. Attention to the subjective experience of subject formation reveals that neoliberal self-making projects can never be complete because they rest on a fundamental lack. The new demands of the subject are articulated not as a positive determination but rather as an open injunction. While the Communist Party in Vietnam provides concrete directions on how to be a good socialist—remember the fatherland, have no more than two children, and so on—no clear guide exists for neoliberal selfhood. Rather, as Žižek (1989) notes, neoliberal imperatives are framed as open injunctions to be free (e.g., "Just be yourself"). However, the differences between these ideals and how people live up to them can be stark. People know they must determine themselves and their happiness on their own, but there is no explicit way for them to do so. With an unclear objective, the self is oriented to a lack with no object to fill it. People have many more options in choosing their own social roles and identities, but this is itself an anxiety-inducing process (Fromm 1941).

Anxiety, then, is what people "feel when the world reveals itself to be caught up in the space between two frames" (Weber 1991, 167). Because these projects rest on a self that requires an object for definition, they are doomed to fail. In turn, this triggers a spiral of worry that people manage by producing industrious subjects and collectives. Neoliberalism thrives on this failure. Because the drive for self-realization has become a responsibility, failure brings not just social disapproval but also self-contempt. In this light, anxiety is both a social practice for becoming a rational, autonomous, and self-governed subject but also evidence of the failure to become that subject. The recursivity of this anxiety plays a powerful role in the production and reproduction of neoliberal subjectivities. Uncertainty about the future may produce intense anxiety, but the future is more ominous still from a perspective that itself is not secure.

Hương, a forty-five-year-old woman, could probably relate to Kiệt's situation in one key way despite her politically favorable family history (lý lịch) and, thus, much different postwar trajectory. The daughter of a high-ranking Party member from Hanoi, she was among the first Vietnamese college students to study in the United States after the normalization of diplomatic relations. Now working in the upper management of a German corporation's offices in Ho Chi Minh City, she and her two children lived in a newly constructed high-rise apartment popular with foreigners (where one of her neighbors was an American psychotherapist, discussed in chapter 5). Yet even with her family connections, she remembered her ten-year-old self constantly scheming to secure basic necessities during the subsidy era. "I had to think (*suy nghĩ*) about [how to do] everything," Hương said, adding in English that "you had to fight tooth and nail just to survive." Conversely, her fourteen-year-old son Quý, who was then vacationing with his cousins in Australia, could not do anything on his own. "No street smarts," she laughed.

Both Hương and Kiệt found it difficult to reconcile the gulf between their and their children's experiences and expectations, and they were not alone. Throughout my fieldwork, members of multiple generations commented on the differences between those who came of age before and after the growth of Vietnam's economy. Of course, people's particular class, age, gender, political affiliation, and family history shape their vantage points on the generation gaps and continue to inflect the course of their lives. Despite the vast array of their perspectives, conversations with Ho Chi Minh City residents often drifted to how older generations managed to sacrifice for the younger ones. Certainly, Hương and Kiệt were grateful that their children would likely never face as much suffering as they had or have to accept such bitter fates. Yet the contemporary promise to determine one's future comes with strings attached. Nam, Quý, and their contemporaries indeed have more options than ever before, but caught between multiple frames they are forced into making more decisions with fewer givens to rely upon, more ambiguous criteria, and less stability and support.

MIDDLE-CLASS ASPIRATIONS AND MORALITIES

With the fastest-growing middle class in Southeast Asia, Vietnam aims to achieve high-middle-income status by 2035, when half its population will have joined the global middle class (World Bank & Ministry of Planning and Investment of Vietnam 2016). Party officials see the path to their ambitious economic target through expanding and supporting an urbanizing middle-class society. Since I began my research, Ho Chi Minh City residents have learned to occupy new spaces of consumerism with greater confidence. Clothing brands and smartphones that seemed out of reach for most of the people I knew ten years ago are now commonplace. Charmingly dilapidated apartment buildings and maze-like alleyways have become crammed with craft beer and cocktail bars, sushi and ramen restaurants, and (of course) cafés that rely more on social media presence than on visibility from the street to attract their clientele. A rumor spread that all buildings under four stories on Thanh Đa, a five-hundred-hectare island in the Saigon River, would be demolished to make way for luxury high-rises, state-of-the-art schools, a new metro line, and even a well-manicured dog park. For many Vietnamese, the rise of the country's middle class is a sign of economic progress but also of widening inequality and environmental degradation (Hansen 2017).

While the impact of the middle class on Ho Chi Minh City's landscape is obvious, defining Vietnam's middle class has proved to be notoriously difficult. Developed for Western populations, standard economic criteria such as household income ignore critical nuances of class formation throughout Southeast Asia (Bélanger et al. 2012). Thus, following Bourdieu (1984), ethnographic analyses of the Vietnamese middle class go beyond purely economic and materialist readings of class to take into account the clusters of practices, aesthetics, and affects that stem from self-consciously middle-class citizenship and lifestyles. For example, the construction of a Vietnamese middle-class identity occurs in relation to creative practices (Taylor 2012; Peters 2012), gender and family (Hoang 2015; Shohet 2017), transportation (Hansen 2017; Earl 2020), and beauty, health, and fitness (Leshkowich 2012; Nguyen Tu 2021), among others. The individuals taking part in them vary widely in terms of standard class markers such as occupation, education, or even income. Thus, the middle class in Ho Chi Minh City is less a distinct segment of the population than a cultural project and negotiation over what it means to be a modern and, increasingly, global citizen (Higgins 2008).[10] This project is rooted in economic trends that have sweeping implications for much of the country, but it is most accessible to those with the skills and technologies to take part in middle-class practices.

The relative economic comfort of the global middle class does not simply shield people from anxiety. Indeed, the construction of the middle class may create new forms of insecurity for Ho Chi Minh City residents. The contemporary abundance of choices, consumer and otherwise, is a distinct break from the subsidy era, when the state supplied people with few options for their daily goods. Today's supermarkets and retail stores give customers dozens of brands to select from and express themselves with. As in reform-era China (McGrath 2008), the everyday imperative to choose confronts people with the fact that their decisions change the future. This, in turn, emphasizes how everyday life is contingent on people's choices and their own responsibility in managing it.[11] The personal stakes of everyday decisions are higher when people believe that they have the ability to fulfill their own desires through a rational assessment of future possibilities. The freedoms and choices made available under *đổi mới* create the conditions for anxiety as individuals must carry "the widespread and unforeseeable implications of one's decision upon [their] shoulders" (Wicks 2009, 211).

New goods and leisure activities may simply pass the time, but they also introduce people to new ideas about personal taste and the difference between the good life and a meaningful one. Ambitions for a particular lifestyle become a project for a desired future self (Elinoff 2012). With so many more options, people both raise their expectations and compare their own selections with those of others. Consumer practices, in turn, become fraught with anxiety over the cultivation of an appropriate taste regime (Arsel and Bean 2013). The expansion of "aspirational horizons" may result in profound anxieties about the good life and what needs to be done in order to attain one (Chua 2014). Furthermore, because the promise and threat of upward and downward mobility, respectively, exist alongside each other for the middle class, people face new insecurities related to the "longing to secure" an increasingly precarious social position (Heiman, Liechty, and Freeman 2012; Stewart 2010). Since Asia's new middle class is legally and economically less protected than the established elite, their economic resources are insufficient to guarantee a respectable place in society (Zhang 2012). The broadening of social practices in constructing middle-classness opens debate on who can legitimately claim a particular status. Hence, the management of middle-class subjectivity across cultural and national boundaries requires constant monitoring and maintenance of one's class identity through the navigation of social boundaries and moral dilemmas.

Moreover, the đổi mới reforms have not erased socialist ideals that hold wealth in suspicion. Its critics charge that the market economy encourages selfish and greedy accumulation and that open-door policies expose the population to Western ideas that undermine long-standing values and relationships (Leshkowich 2014a). Thus, new consumer products and services are the source of both newfound pleasures and an ethical ambivalence about them (Jellema 2005). Many Ho Chi Minh City residents accuse Vietnam's new superrich of attaining their extravagant wealth through corruption and exploitation. Conversely, the middle class balance their new lifestyles with prudent morality—at least according to those who consider themselves to be in their ranks. The pressure to maintain one's own moral standing in ethically ambiguous terrain often leads people to reaffirm gender and family norms that are foundational to moral personhood in Vietnam (Trinh 2022). Of course, Ho Chi Minh City's middle class does not hold a monopoly on anxiety, as worries about appropriate consumption, underachievement, and missed opportunities also extend beyond the fringes of the middle class. Perhaps what most characterizes the anxieties of the upwardly mobile, then, is how they emerge in relation to aspirations toward particular ways of being in the world associated with middle-class lifestyles. Working toward them becomes a project of self and class-making that increasingly rely on skills and technologies associated with the psy-disciplines.

BEYOND THE CLINIC

During the first few months of the COVID-19 pandemic, when much of the world was in lockdown and people with shortened attention spans sought out both distraction and mental health support, therapist influencers gained a foothold across social media platforms. Following the mold of wellness influencers who dispense advice on diet and exercise, these famous-on-the-internet psychotherapists promote a kind of emotional fitness. Due to the successful containment of the coronavirus, Vietnam enjoyed a relative degree of normality during the first eighteen months of the pandemic, but the arrival of the more infectious Delta variant in the spring of 2021 sent much of the country into lockdown. Popular interest in mental health, especially among young people, soared. The most well known of Vietnam's therapist influencers is a twenty-three-year-old teacher and counselor at an international school in Hanoi[12] named Đinh Ngọc Bình, who operates under the username @ngocbinhtamly (Ngọc Bình Psychology) and boasts more than 260,000 followers on TikTok, a short-form video sharing app. Sporting his trademark oversized eyeglasses and a pearl necklace, he addresses a wide range of mental health topics of interest to his fellow "Gen Zers" (people born between the late 1990s and the 2010s), including emotional intelligence (*trí tuệ cảm xúc*), parental conflicts and pressures, toxic relationships (*MQH* [*mối quan hệ*] *toxic*), and career paths in psychology.

In most of his posts, Ngọc Bình speaks directly into the camera as if the viewer were one of his clients. For a video on how to reduce stress (*strés* or *căng thẳng*), he suggests concentrating on your bodily sensations, breathing, and footsteps.[13] These tips are derived from the mindfulness meditation practices made famous in the West by the Vietnamese monk Thích Nhất Hạnh, but no reference to their Buddhist origins is made in the video. Ngọc Bình's final suggestion for decreasing tension—reserving time to do something you like—coincides with footage of him shopping for brand-name basketball shoes. Another TikTok is set to the trending sound of a selection from the song "Choices (Yup)" by the American West Coast rapper E-40.[14] As in other video posts with the same audio track, Ngọc Bình points to text appearing on screen, nodding his head in disapproval or smiling and giving a thumbs up to the words *nope* and *yup*, in time with the music. This video, in particular, is on the "do's and don'ts" of depression. The "nopes" to avoid include drinking alcohol, pretending to be optimistic, and diagnosing yourself with depression, among other maladaptive strategies. The "yups" are writing down one's sorrow, accepting one's sadness, and talking about it with a close friend or a professional. The warning about self-diagnosing and the prompt to consult a psychotherapist underscore the field's professional expertise. A major theme throughout his posts is the importance of embracing all of the emotions in life, not just the positive, prosocial ones. As an unofficial ambassador of psychotherapy in Vietnam, Ngọc Bình raises awareness of the intellectual and emotional tools of psychology that help people understand not just themselves but others as well (Chi Mai 2022).

Ngọc Bình's rise to fame is part of an emerging "psycho-boom" (Kleinman 2010) across East and Southeast Asia. Popular interest not just in psychiatry and psychotherapy but also in self-help literature, lifestyle coaching, and inspirational videos, memes, and marketing campaigns shared on social media reflects a growing industry of self-interest (Yang 2014; Zhang 2014). Mental health workers have grown in force: school counselors, speech and language pathologists, and advanced behavioral analysts, in addition to psychotherapists and psychiatrists.

The vocabulary of madness (điên rồ), too, has proliferated to include biomedical terms such as *stress* (*strés*), *depression* (*trầm cảm*), and *autism* (*tự kỷ*).[15] The new understandings of the inner self that are being used by many people—not just mental health professionals—as the basis for reimagining one's self and its place in the world are critical to the psycho-boom's market in Vietnam (Tran 2017). The cultivation and aesthetic appreciation of one's own interiority constructs the self as a modern individual (i.e., one who self-consciously defies feudal traditions and collective definitions of the self in favor of self-determination). Once deemed too abstract, psychological concepts about emotion, self-esteem, and unconscious desires have seeped into everyday conversation. Advocates of the turn toward the psychological claim that it is only to be expected. Echoing Maslow's hierarchy of needs,[16] their argument posits that the relative ease with which people's physical needs are fulfilled in the reform era allows them to focus their energies on their emotional ones.

However, changing economic tides cannot wholly account for the inward turn that has become a hallmark of neoliberal economies. Self-discovery is not a natural process, but rather must be learned. Increasingly, people are taught to discover themselves with conceptual tools from the professional fields of knowledge related to the workings of the mind that Nikolas Rose terms the *psy-disciplines*. In the West, the psy-disciplines compel individuals to make everyday life a project of the self and give them the tools to reinvent the self. People are meant to work on their emotions, spousal relations, and affective labor in the workplace and cultivate a lifestyle that maximizes their own existence to themselves (Rose 1992). The late-capitalist demand for soft skills depends on forms of psychological expertise in school and workplace environments, and increasingly those skills are being taken home (Hochschild 1983; Illouz 2008). Furthermore, methods to maximize self-efficiency draw from psychotherapeutic techniques. For example, in addition to private psychotherapy sessions, many counseling centers in Vietnam offer seminars on conflict resolution to teams at businesses and schools. Together, therapeutic culture and neoliberal entrepreneurialism posit the individual as the site of healing and self-making as well as of economic development and personal alienation (Freeman 2014; Duncan 2018).

Perhaps nowhere are the characteristics of the self-sufficient, individuated neoliberal subject cultivated and naturalized so well as in the clinic (Rose 2006; Furedi 2004), and critics of biomedical psychiatry and its global spread charge that the field naturalizes neoliberal ideas of selfhood under the guise of healing. Indeed, psychological research that focuses on psychological phenomena independent of their cultural and historical context both reflects and reinforces neoliberal ideals that posit a radical distinction between self and society (Adams et al. 2019). The Western discourse of psychiatry is not only used to introduce new ideas about feelings and behavior but also to regulate them for political and economic gain

(Ecks 2016). For example, the recent movement for global mental health has largely gained traction by highlighting the negative impacts of psychiatric distress on economic productivity, not just physical health (Patel 2014). The Lancet Commission on Global Mental Health and Sustainable Development (Patel et al. 2018) estimated that the global mental health crisis will cost $16 trillion by 2030. Mental health concerns have also taken center stage in recent years at the World Bank, the United Nations General Assembly, and the Davos Forum. Public health-oriented research on the burden of mental illness in non-Western contexts often addresses the lack of proper mental health literacy among the most vulnerable of populations and the need to educate health care workers and patients about proper mental health care. However, to what end would addressing the "mental health gap" between those who need treatment and those who receive it actually benefit people in the Global South (Rose 2019)? Has the rise of biomedical psychiatry, often at the expense of local ways of understanding and treating mental illness, led to a new form of medical imperialism (Summerfield 2008)?

While the conceptual framework of neoliberal subject formation does have considerable explanatory power, it does not adequately account for the ambivalences and contradictions that psy-discipline's advocates—experts and laypersons alike—often experience with these new technologies of the self. Despite the power of global mental health's new ways of imagining the self, they do not replace local understandings of moral selfhood. After all, Ngọc Bình's videos stress the use of emotional intelligence in service of understanding oneself and others. Cường, a twenty-four-year-old graduate student, was drawn to clinical psychology because, according to him, he struggled to understand himself and communicate with his family. He found in his studies the means to get into another person's perspective, which he would need to bridge the gap in experience and perspective between him and his parents, who suffered staggering family losses and personal injuries during and after the war. According to Cường, their conception of a good life emphasizes stability and safety over the meaning and passion he desired for his own career. For him, psychology is a tool for better enacting filial piety. The desire to communicate himself better to his parents reflects a need for their validation, which runs against neoliberal ideals of self-sufficiency and autonomy. Indeed, emerging forms of psychiatric practice may also generate therapeutic sites of sociality, not just individuality, to contest such projects and comment on their failures (Duncan 2017).

The concept of psy-sociality frames global mental health practices as a means of governance and healing (Duncan 2017; Matza 2018). New individual identities and social formations have emerged from an expertise of the mind and a community of emotional pain (Duncan 2018). Psy-sociality foregrounds the social connections that are remade in the wake of the neoliberalization of everyday life. Despite the glaring hegemonic imposition of Western concepts of personhood and emotion implied in the globalization of biomedical psychiatry, patients and practitioners alike find that much of these regimes of knowledge resonates with their own experiences. In spaces of conflict and contradiction, people transform both themselves and these technologies of the self as they negotiate competing visions of a good and moral life. Imagining new potentials and limits for one's life requires a realignment of existing ones, and attending to this process provides insight into the pleasures and perils of the psy-disciplines.

Although the psychotherapeutic turn may seem limited to a small but growing community of disciples, it has far-reaching implications for contemporary Vietnamese society. If new landscapes of the psychological alter the horizon of the political (Matza 2018), shifting configurations of the mind and heart shape ongoing debates over not just what it means to be happy and healthy, but also what it means to be true to yourself or to be a Vietnamese citizen. Ho Chi Minh City residents use the psy-disciplines to make sense of not only themselves but also the current historical moment. Since ideas about the self are intertwined with different forms of anxiety, new models of the self occasion new forms of anxiety. *A Life of Worry* takes the presence of anxiety as something that is not simply good or bad, normal or abnormal, or healthy or pathological. Dichotomies that implicitly frame anxiety as something that prevents well-being rely on a medicalized logic of self-maximization. Rather, anxiety is evidence of people's struggles with reconciling the conflicting demands of the individual and the social.

THE BEST-LAID PLANS

On January 1, 2007, I arrived in Ho Chi Minh City to study the long-term impacts of war on mental health with several topics to explore and methods to deploy, very few of which would actually prove useful. One of these was to construct a cultural taxonomy of emotions. Doing so would identify the dominant feelings of the reform era and allow for comparisons across historical periods. Research participants would be asked to do a pile sort exercise in which they read through a list of items and then group them into categories. Thus, the first step of my data collection was to generate an inventory of different emotions (*cảm xúc*, a term I explore further in chapter 3). My plan was to simply ask a wide range of people to name various examples of emotions. How hard could it be?

Several months and bureaucratic hurdles later, my research assistant Vũng and I, guided by representatives from a local ward's people's committee, finally set out with pen and paper to conduct a free list exercise. When Vũng asked if we should collect data only from people with a college degree, he explained that only the most educated people would be able to complete the activity. I dismissed his concern. Why would people with less education be unable to identify various feelings? Given that educational levels are often used as a proxy for socioeconomic status in Vietnam, focusing only on college graduates would skew the sample to the upper class. Of course, Vũng's prediction was right. College graduates seemed to enjoy the task. I often noted a wry smile on their faces as they came up with items for the free list: happiness (*vui*) and satisfaction (*hài lòng*), sadness/boredom (*buồn*) and gloominess (*u sầu*), anger (*giận dữ*) and jealousy (*ghen tuông*), lovestruck (*phải lòng*) and lovesick (*thất tình*), and maudlin (*ướt át*). One of my favorite entries, *phê*, from the word *cà phê* (coffee), refers to a state of passion and flow when engrossed by a new work of art or a favorite pastime and physiologically resembles the buzz of caffeine. Meanwhile, people with less education often struggled to produce more than a handful of examples. Many were confused by the term *emotions*, so we tried a number of synonyms—including "psychological sentiments" (*tình cảm tâm lý*), "joys and sorrows" (*vui buồn*), and the classifiers for negative and positive emotions (*nỗi niềm*)—to little avail. Others wrote down types of relationships, such as wife and husband (*vợ chồng*) or mother and child (*má con*). What began as an attempt to identify the range of emotions that epitomizes the contemporary moment instead found that perhaps the very concept of emotion itself is indicative of an emergent subjectivity.

Clearly, I had to go back to the drawing board. During these long stretches of free time at the beginning of fieldwork, I frequented a sidewalk café consisting of plastic tables and stools that were moved throughout the day to follow the shade of my apartment complex. Each time I went there, I resolved not to go back upstairs until I had thought through a logistical challenge in my research or at least reached some new insight into it, sometimes ordering a second cup of *cà phê sữa đá* (iced coffee with condensed milk) to keep me alert. The more I did this, however, the worse my problems seemed to get, and I often found myself in a panic—heart racing, hands shaking, thinking catastrophic—over my research. This was not the *phê* of an intellectual breakthrough. I did not realize at the time that a *cà phê sữa đá* is much stronger than the brewed coffee I drank in the United States—the robusta beans grown in Vietnam have twice as much caffeine as the arabica beans that are more common in the rest of the world. Did I panic because of a genuine concern over my research or because of a *cà phê sữa đá*? Of course, both factors played a role at the sidewalk café. Anthropologists have long been drawn to the study of emotion because of this interplay between the embodied and the interpretive. Robert Levy (1984) argued that emotions are a subset of physical feelings that are attributed to causes external to the body. When people believe that these sensations come from within the body, they often label them as some form of illness. Thus, when I assumed that my heartbeat and thoughts were racing because of fieldwork problems, I labeled them anxiety—which I tried to overcome by persevering with more coffee. When I belatedly realized I was also ingesting unhealthy amounts of caffeine, the same problem had the opposite solution. This book is less invested in the question of whether or not my alarm—or anyone else's—was "real" than in exploring how people determine the presence of anxiety when they experience it themselves or encounter it among others. As my changing interpretations of those bouts of panic demonstrate, emotions are partly constructed by how they are perceived. Bated breath, dilated pupils, and a rapid heartbeat are signs of anxiety in relation to an expected outcome that is bleak, but those same bodily states can be experienced as excitement in a more optimistic mode. The manner in which Ho Chi Minh City residents come to classify physical, mental, and social states as one emotion or another impacts their understanding and experience of themselves as emotional beings.

How people assess their anxiety is not just a theoretical question but a methodological one as well. Throughout the book, I chronicle how Ho Chi Minh City residents gauge, control, expel, avoid, sublimate, and give in to their anxieties. This documentation does not simply provide a voyeuristic perspective into the worried minds of the Vietnamese. Indeed, no objective method of collecting or analyzing data on anxiety (or anything else for that matter) exists in the anthropological tool kit. Because researchers' subject positions mediate their observations and interpretations, deep empathy is not enough to transcend the differences between various frameworks on anxiety. The analytical task at hand, then, is not to transcend these affective filters. Translating them has the benefit of contextualizing the emotions, but we should not be so naive as to believe that a translation thorough enough can yield mutual understanding. As biomedical theories of anxiety increasingly gain professional stature and widespread acceptance in Vietnam, the power differences between the various models of emotion, affect, and sentiment mask points of contention and conflict. I had to be highly aware of my own filters and biases through which I interpret anxiety, and I invite readers to do the same. Thus, this research and this book, the product of that research, is an intersubjective achievement (Throop 2010) in which we will encounter experiences that resonate with our own life story. Yet, like a certain kitchen half a world away, the context of these strangely familiar feelings is different, and that context makes all the difference.

Developing an interpersonal model of anxiety recognizes that relationships can be a powerful medium of anxiety. Ho Chi Minh City residents often process emotional experiences in a relational idiom (see chapters 2 and 3). For them, worry emerges from and functions as part of people's connections with family and friends, neighbors and fellow citizens, and a visiting anthropologist, among others. Indeed, how my interlocutors and I related to each other may have influenced their own reflections on the emotions. Interviewing techniques such as actively listening, probing, and following up coincide with expressions of concern that implicated me in the mutual relations of care that define worry in Vietnam. (Of course, these are not mutually exclusive!) In life history and person-centered ethnographic interviews with a wide range of Ho Chi Minh City residents, my interlocutors and I explored their emotional lives as I invited them to reflect on themselves. Some said they did not often get these opportunities, mentioning fear of judgment, gossip, or unsolicited advice from their usual social circles. They used our conversations to mull over and experiment with emerging ideas about the emotions, mental health, and the good life.

Furthermore, relational components of ethnographic methods are tied to the researchers' own positionality. Calling for a reflexive dialogue about the racial, gender, and class dynamics that underpin research methodologies, Hoang (2015) notes that her identity as a Vietnamese American researcher gave her insider access on a temporary basis while marking her as a permanent outsider. Upon learning I was an American-born child of Vietnamese refugees, many Ho Chi Minh City residents told me that their "dream" (they used the English word) was to visit or even move to the United States. Many detailed, often with a bitter laugh, their failed attempts to "cross the sea" (*vượt biển*) during the subsidy era. The United States loomed large in their imagination as a proverbial land of milk and honey and the pinnacle of modernity to which they aspired. Responding to some of my questions and probes about their personal experiences, people occasionally asked me, in return, what an American would do in their situation, or framed their answers explicitly in apologetic and self-deprecating terms of how they understood the differences between Vietnamese and American culture. The self-Orientalizing manner in which my interlocutors dichotomized West from East, and modern from traditional, should not be taken at face value, but rather should be understood as a heuristic device for making sense of the changes in their own surroundings.

The clearest articulations of new ways of worrying in Ho Chi Minh City are to be found at the psychiatric clinic and, increasingly, in psychotherapeutic offices. My clinical ethnography was based at the Ho Chi Minh City Psychiatric Hospital outpatient clinic as well as at Army Hospital 175 in Ho Chi Minh City and the National Psychiatric Hospital II in Biên Hoà in neighboring Đồng Nai Province. Most of my time was spent with patients as they made their way through the hospitals' complex bureaucratic system, but I also interviewed and observed doctors, nurses, and hospital administrators. During my initial research trips to Ho Chi Minh City, examining nonpharmaceutical treatments for mental health problems was difficult, given the dearth of psychotherapeutic services. The following decade, however, saw a burgeoning industry of private counseling centers that I documented by interviewing therapists and clients and attending training courses, workshops, and networking events for local and foreign psy-experts, including special education teachers, speech and language pathologists, and recent Vietnamese college graduates returning from their studies abroad with degrees in psychology that they hoped to parlay into careers in psychotherapy.

Tracing the extent of the reach of the psy-disciplines requires us to expand our analytical focus to everyday spaces of work and leisure in Ho Chi Minh City. To explore the less clearly demarcated area of the evolving emotional life of Ho Chi Minh City's middle class, I initially relied on snowball sampling from a small number of research contacts. Eventually, this network expanded widely, as many of the participants generously facilitated the research because they found the topic to be *hay* (interesting). When possible, I met with people in their homes in order to observe the household dynamics. However, these dynamics also prevented insightful individual interviews, as multigenerational homes came with significant interruptions. Given that the city's public spaces provide more privacy than crowded households, individual interviews were usually conducted at cafés. Going to new cafés is a popular pastime in Ho Chi Minh City, which has a thriving café culture ranging from simple sidewalk cafés to brick-and-mortar establishments with opulent gardens and rooftop terraces. These "third spaces," separate from the home and the workplace, offer opportunities to explore new ideas and experiment with new identities. Here, the interviews could blend in with the social outings, business meetings, and study sessions happening around us. Critically, this anonymity allowed me to interview women, as meeting in a private home risks accusations of impropriety from ever-present neighbors.

Part 1 of this book examines the resources people use to make sense of anxious experiences. At the heart of why I had problems with the free-list exercise in the first place was my assumption that emotions were a category of everyday experience relevant to most Ho Chi Minh City residents. Indeed, as much as Westerners take the emotions as a bedrock of shared human experience, this notion varied in Vietnam. While every person I met in Ho Chi Minh City believed that some kind of affective process is critical to one's humanity in general as well as to one's identity in particular, what these processes look like and their implications for understanding anxiety differ along fault lines of class, gender, and generation. While this chapter provides an overview of academic theories of anxiety, chapter 2 explores how Ho Chi Minh City residents understand it. For them, anxiety and worry are forms of moral sentiment that connect people through gendered relations of care. (Notions of sentiment are predicated on ideals of a relational selfhood, hence the free-list entries of social relationships.) Worrying for someone puts an individual in a relationship marked by an acknowledgment of their vulnerability and a concern for their well-being. Chapter 3 explores an alternative discourse of emotion and selfhood emerging among Ho Chi Minh City's upwardly mobile. The categories of sentiment and emotion are not simply empty vessels of affective experience. The shape that people give to an amorphous experience like anxiety impacts how it is experienced, interpreted, and acted upon. Whether anxiety is interpreted through the lens of a moral sentiment or an emotion reflects a class position in the context of increasing economic inequality. Ho Chi Minh City's middle class has found in the emotions a new way of being-in-the-world. Together, chapters 2 and 3 document the perhaps futile attempts to pin down anxiety, that most inchoate and free-floating of experiences.

Part 2 focuses on one of anxiety's most extreme manifestations: mental illness. Critics of biomedical psychiatry argue that the clinic naturalizes the self-sufficient, individuated neoliberal subject by medicalizing emotional distress. However, I disentangle this process by demonstrating that the medicalization (chapter 4) and psychologization (chapter 5) of anxiety are distinct processes in Vietnam. Whether people receive psychopharmaceutical or psychotherapeutic treatments, they are taught to focus on the problematic emotion itself instead of on the physical symptoms of mental illnesses or the social situations that give rise to them. Patients at the Ho Chi Minh City Psychiatric Hospital are encouraged to identify anxiety as the ultimate target of intervention instead of the headaches and insomnia that brought them to the hospital, and clients undergoing cognitive behavioral therapy learn to identify triggering situations and label their reactions to them as anxiety. If new landscapes of the psychological alter the horizon of the political, shifting configurations of the mind and heart shape ongoing debates over not just what it means to be happy and healthy but also what it means to be your authentic self or a Vietnamese citizen.

However, part 2 also illuminates how engagement with biomedical treatments such as psychopharmaceuticals (chapter 4) and psychotherapy (chapter 5) may generate new forms of sociality, not just the turn inward that many critics predict. Although these treatments are designed to promote the neoliberal ideal of self-governance, the psy-turn also lays the foundation for alternative regimes of selfhood (Matza 2018; Duncan 2018; Zhang 2020). The experience of Ho Chi Minh City residents with the psy-disciplines cautions against dismissing them as altogether apolitical. Instead, these experiences shift the criteria of what counts as political. People use ideas rooted in psychotherapeutic models of anxiety to critique the limits placed on their lives and rethink the possibilities for themselves and their families (Pritzker and Duncan 2019). Indeed, new understandings of the emotions in general provide clients a third-person perspective on themselves, their loved ones, and their communities through richly embodied experiences of relating to others.

Part 3 inverts many of the themes of part 1. Instead of analyzing how anxiety is articulated by social roles, discourses, and institutions, these chapters focus on how anxiety itself is a socially productive force to be reckoned with. I return to the supposed futilities of understanding anxiety as sentiment or emotion to examine them not as limitations but rather as motivation for social action. Moving beyond the clinic, chapter 6 investigates what happens when Ho Chi Minh City residents apply new ideas about the self and emotion to their own lives. People are not always in control of the technologies of the self they use in their romantic self-making projects. Whether by choice or by force, people find themselves in predicaments that effectively shake the rug from underneath them. Figuring out the simple question of what they want out of life calls for a major reconsideration of their priorities. When it comes to matters of the heart, attempts to be a modern subject may create an anxiety about the self that gets (mis)labeled as love. Chapter 7 concludes the book by asking what Vietnam's age of anxiety has to teach us as a new, global age of anxiety takes shape. I propose an agenda for ethnographic research on anxiety and anxiety disorders. Establishing a cross-cultural framework will help us better appreciate the workings of anxiety and social processes together. I focus most on anxiety's links between the personal and the political. A constant yet unidentifiable sense of unease is not an objective fact but rather something that is cultivated. However, anxiety does not just have dangers and vulnerabilities but also offers new potential for a different kind of politics based on care.

2

Moral Sentiments

When I met Hoa, a twenty-six-year-old woman, for the first time in five years, she gave me a hug—back then a rare greeting in Vietnam. Her time in the United States, I thought, had changed her. Hoa's cheery demeanor and expressive speech—now peppered with colloquialisms from the American South, as we caught up at a café near her brother's house in Gò Vấp District—were a striking contrast to the last time we had met, on an afternoon about a month before she moved to the United States. She had told me, like it was a secret, of a dread that grew as her departure date approached. Her older sister had recently married an American man she had met online, and her parents had decided that Hoa was to join her sister in Georgia to keep her company and help with any future children. Hoa was also to study to become a pharmacist (even though she had nearly completed her degree requirements in economics). At this point, Hoa believed there was no turning back, as all of the paperwork had been completed, tickets bought, and money borrowed. When I expressed my gratitude for her significant help with my research, she teared up and waved goodbye before quickly turning down Lê Thánh Tôn Street to her bus stop.

Much did change for Hoa when she moved to the United States. Initially, she struggled with language barriers, making new friends, and a sense of homesickness and dislocation. A few months later, her father suddenly died of a stroke, but her mother and sister kept his death from her, out of fear that she would return permanently to Ho Chi Minh City to be with her mother. She discovered the news only when her cousin expressed his condolences to her in a WhatsApp message. Forbidden from returning home for her father's funeral, Hoa persevered and eventually received a bachelor's degree in chemistry from a prestigious university, found work as a pharmacy technician, and had recently become engaged herself. She adored her nephew and enjoyed spending time with her new friends and traveling within the United States.

During this first trip back to Vietnam for her, Hoa spent most of her free time at her brother's house or in nearby Đồng Nai Province, where she grew up. Because she had yet to see the dramatic changes in the city's downtown known as District 1, we decided to go to the newly opened pedestrian walkway on Nguyễn Huệ Street. What was supposed to be a quick stop at her brother's house for Hoa to get a motorbike helmet dragged on when Giang, her fifty-six-year-old mother, came downstairs. She asked Hoa if she needed any spending money and gave her some anyway when she said no. Then Giang asked me if I was hungry. I said no, but she brought out a tray of candied ginger and coconut for me anyway. Before we could leave, she gave some more money to Hoa, who happily protested.

WORRY AS A SOCIAL PRACTICE

Anxiety and worry take many forms in Hoa's story: her fear of the unknown in the United States, separation and social anxiety, economic risks, self-imposed and family expectations, and concern over the fate of loved ones. However, they are also present in the way Giang pressed money into her daughter's hand and asked if I had eaten yet. Finally on our way to District 1, I commented to Hoa on how much her mother doted on her. I thought she was going to say, "She cares about me," but instead she said, "She worries about me." The sentiment was not far off. Giang's actions can also be interpreted as displays of maternal affection, politeness, and generosity, but in Vietnam they occupy much of the same conceptual terrain as worry.

In everyday conversations in Vietnam, anxiety and worry carry a wide range of meanings that are interrelated but shift in emphasis according to context. First, not dissimilar to its predominant understanding in the West, worry (lo, lo lắng) can refer to the negatively charged mental activity that allocates cognitive resources toward the preparation of some task or the defense against a potentially unpleasant experience. Indeed, thinking and worrying can be used interchangeably, including in the psychiatric discourses discussed in chapter 4.[1] With its orientation toward an unknown future, worry is a form of imagination that links creative potential and political structure and leads to social action (Appadurai 1996; McMullin and Dao 2014). In an analysis of selective reproduction technologies in Hanoi, Gammeltoft (2014) suggests that anthropological analysis of the imaginary sheds light on the implicit yet influential moods and sensations at the convergence of subjective experience and political power. Second, worry is often discussed in behavioral terms, usually related to managing tasks, chores, and responsibilities. For example, people who can worry for themselves (tự lo) are praised for their independence and initiative. Conversely, people who do not know how to worry (không biết lo) are deemed feckless and irresponsible. In this context, worry is a positively valued indication that a person is competent, savvy, and able to take care of others instead of requiring that others take care of them. Within a cosmology of everyday life as a series of tasks that must be resolved, the discourse of worry imbues even the most banal sources of anxiety with moral weight. Finally, and most germane to Hoa and Giang, *worry* also describes the social obligation to care for others. Feelings of concern bring people into relationships based on an acknowledged vulnerability and indebtedness that shape the social roles and expectations of those involved (Shohet 2021). Such enactments of worry are differently used as a means to forge and strengthen emotional relations to others vis-à-vis notions of sentiment. This makes it difficult to distinguish between the object of worry and the process of worry itself.

This chapter examines how Ho Chi Minh City residents make sense of all of these anxious states, gestures, and relationships in relation to morality and modernity. The everyday experience of worrying and being worried for in Vietnam is articulated in terms of everyday care and concern, family roles and obligations, and moral sentiments. Situated within assessments of gendered morality, Vietnamese discourses of anxiety emphasize the relations of sentiment (*tình cảm*) between individuals and the object of their care. The existentially fraught experience of focusing on life's uncertainties becomes a moral virtue when directed toward another person. Anxiety, then, is a matter of "worrying-for" as well as "worrying-about." For women especially, worry is a burden that is to be cultivated and endured as matters of social obligation and moral virtue. This was often portrayed as a timeless exemplar of Vietnamese culture in the way Ho Chi Minh City residents explained their understandings of worry to me, and many of these conversations veered toward essentialist tropes about gender and traditional values. These ideals may seem well-defined, but how people attempt (and often fail) to live up to them reveals a far murkier picture of morality. Moreover, as the *đổi mới* era has left so much of Vietnamese social life in flux, new opportunities arise for moral behavior and breakdown. Shifting models of anxiety presage new approaches to moral dilemmas. In the context of profound social changes, many communities may experience a society-wide moral breakdown (Robbins 2004; Zigon 2007).

Understanding how anxiety and related emotional states are configured through ethical modes of being and relating starts with the recognition that our affective, bodily, and ethical dispositions are entangled with others (Geurts 2002; Csordas 2008; Stevenson 2014; Mattingly 2014; Throop 2014). Attending to anxiety's relational qualities challenges the common assumption that it is fundamentally a private experience. When most Vietnamese discuss their and each other's anxiety, they delve into the complications of social relationships more often than the depths of feelings. However, while anxiety can be shaped and patterned by social institutions and discourses, it cannot be reduced to them. That is, our existence as humans is "at once excessive, uncertain, and emergent" (Mattingly and Throop 2018, 482). Grounding anxiety in social interactions and practices, I examine how affective experiences become a site of ethical reasoning and bring ethnographic data on gendered forms of care to bear on anthropological theories of morality.

People's understandings of the emotional inform their sense of the social, and emotions function partly as a critical discourse through which social relations are negotiated (Lutz 1982). Culturally specific models of anxiety provide people with the frameworks to interpret their worries and to help them order their lives. Thus, the emotions of expectation, whether positive in the case of hope or negative in the case of anxiety, are not only cognitive schemas but also "politically charged dramas that shape the rhythms of activity and the experiences and expectations of participants" (Mattingly 2010, 43). Because the experience of anxiety and the construction of the self are intertwined, how people understand anxiety cannot be separated from notions of self and personhood.

For example, the biological, psychological, and philosophical theories of anxiety so prevalent in Western understandings reflect a monadic orientation to selfhood in which the inner self is conceptualized as radically distinct from its external environment. Here, selfhood is generally considered to be contained within an integrated locus of thought, emotion, and personal responsibility (Shweder and Bourne 1984). Western theories of emotion emphasize a linear process that consists of a biophysical force (Lakoff and Johnson 1980). This is reflected in how psychologists typically distinguish between anxiety, stress, and worry. Worry manifests as thoughts caused by concerns and uncertainties about the future. In other words, it is an attempt to solve a problem mentally. Stress is the physiological response to these uncertainties. Experienced at both a bodily and a cognitive level, anxiety is the affective combination of worry and stress. The dichotomy between individual experience and social interaction prevents an understanding of anxiety and worry as an intersubjective phenomenon, an emotional exchange between individuals, or a sociopolitical condition.

In Vietnamese, however, the semantic distinction between anxiety and worry is not made. Relying on a relational orientation to selfhood, the Vietnamese discourse of worry emphasizes anxiety as both a form of social action and an interpersonal relationship. That is, anxiety and worry are understood not just as a private feeling but also as one that connects people to each other. Mediating the construction of moral personhood, cultural models of worry help people understand themselves as good children, parents, friends, and so on (Tran 2017). The answer to the question of who worries in Vietnam does not point primarily to a particular personality type like the neurotic. Rather, an analysis of anxiety's relation to personhood reveals its moral character.

SELF AND SENTIMENT

During my visits in her kitchen, Bác Lan often asked to practice her English with me. Like many people of her generation, socioeconomic status, and educational background, her English featured a noticeable French accent. Although past the age at which most women in Vietnam are made by law to retire (fifty-five years), she hoped that improved English skills would be useful in potential side business ventures. The following exchange, in which she described a long-ago trip to Paris to visit her sister, comes from one of our impromptu English lessons:

AT: What do you remember about Europe?

BL: The houses [buildings] are very tall. The streets are very long, very wide. Everything is beautiful and clean.

AT: What about the people?

BL: *Cái suy nghĩ là gì, con?* (How do you say "*suy nghĩ*"?)

AT: Their thinking or mentality.

BL: Ah, *mentalité*. Their *mentalité* is real [realistic/pragmatic].[2] They think about money and work.

AT: What do Vietnamese people think about?

BL: Emotion.

AT: "Emotion" *bằng tiếng Việt là gì?* (What is "emotion" in Vietnamese?)

BL: *Tình cảm.*

Tình cảm is a core concept through which people in Vietnam organize their lives and their identities. It has previously been translated as *emotion* (Rydstrøm 2003; Gammeltoft 1999), as *interactive sensibility* (Bayly 2020), as *affection* (Leshkowich 2014a), and as *love, care, and concern* (Shohet 2018). Although such conceptualizations certainly overlap, I propose understanding *tình cảm* through the lens of sentiment to explore how anxiety and selfhood are used to define each other in Vietnam, because it emphasizes intersubjectivity. Although *tình cảm* semantically includes the general category of the emotions (see chapter 3), it is discussed primarily in terms of an emotional attachment to someone. For example, a forty-seven-year-old woman explained to me that while the English language had only the word *love*, Vietnamese had two separate words: *tình yêu* (romantic love) and *tình cảm* (platonic love). Examples include the type of sentiments shared by parents and children, teachers and students, and fellow citizens with each other. As Thuận, a twenty-two-year-old man, told me, *tình cảm* is one's own subjective commentary (*nhận xét chủ quan*) on another person. Thus, sentiment forms the indexical basis on which people interact with each other and understand themselves and their relationship with the world around them.

Tình cảm refers not just to one's own emotions but to those collective feelings. It is considered to be inherently prosocial and moral. For example, negative feelings toward someone else (e.g., hate or jealousy) are not classified as *tình cảm* but rather as merely one's opinions about that person. Thus, *tình cảm* contributes to the relational character of Vietnamese selfhood, which is defined not in opposition to the world but instead in relation to its social, physical, and supernatural surroundings. Throughout my interviews, hypothetical examples of emotions that were not about another person were rare. That notions of *tình cảm* strongly imply that its object is a person underscores its distinctness from Western understandings of emotion as a stand-alone category of individual feeling states. The sentimental self is a matrix of sociomoral relations to be cultivated and evaluated through other people.

According to Ho Chi Minh City residents, sentiment is so important because it fosters social relationships that are based on mutual interdependence and an ethical orientation to others. Enduring and harmonious relations are produced through "the continual affirmation of the value of *tình cảm*" (Shohet 2021). In their discussions of how sentiment is expressed, my interlocutors described both affective and material forms of care, especially inquiring (*hỏi thăm*, lit. visiting and asking) after people and their loved ones and providing material resources and support such as small, routine gifts or lending money to friends and family. Sharing in the joys and sorrows (*vui buồn*, which is also a general term for the emotions) of others is the grist of much of Vietnamese social life. Asking someone to send their respects to a third party is not a mere formality or pleasantry, as it is expected that those respects will be relayed. Demonstrating *tình cảm* requires an intimate understanding of proper decorum and a range of virtues, including respect, conscientiousness, and self-denial, in order to navigate the bustle of everyday social interactions with minimal confrontations (Shohet 2013).

Moral behavior requires the acceptance of the social role one occupies as prescribed by Vietnamese neo-Confucianism. A hierarchical and, to a lesser extent, mutual mode of emotional investment between lords and subjects as well as parents and children characterizes what Haiyan Lee (2007) describes as the "Confucian structure of feeling." Similar to Mauss's (1990) notion of the gift, sentiment facilitates reciprocity and sociality, and to reject a gift risks a loss of social and moral standing for all parties involved. The maxim *sống có tình có nghĩa* (When you live, you have sentiment and responsibility) highlights how affection/compassion (*tình thương*) for and responsibility (*nghĩa vụ*) and indebtedness to others are the foundation of stable, long-term, and meaningful relationships. Transgressions can range from trivial to dramatic. For example, Sơn, a twenty-nine-year-old man, recalled to me watching with equal parts fascination and contempt as a group of Canadian tourists paid for each of their own desserts at an ice cream parlor. He was even tempted to pay the tab on their behalf so that he could avoid witnessing what he admitted was a petty infraction of proper sentiment. Of course, extreme economic matters are cause for more concern as the moral economy of sentiment imbues interpersonal relationships.

Sentiment does not reside within an individual but rather circulates among individuals. Displays of sentiment that adhere to proper decorum across a wide range of situations demonstrate one's intimate understanding of the virtues necessary to navigate the melee of hierarchical social interactions (Shohet 2021). Smooth, nonconfrontational sociality requires constant attention, accommodation, and adjustment to others. As a key force behind moral action, sentiment becomes embodied in and through practices that are rooted in specific social situations and interpersonal histories (Shohet 2021). Foregrounding the social and intersubjective quality of *tình cảm*, Rydstrøm (2003a) argues that villagers in Vietnam's Red River Delta are not concerned with the authenticity of the emotions so long as they are expressed in a contextually appropriate manner. However, the people I knew in Ho Chi Minh City often questioned the sincerity of someone's *tình cảm*, possibly reflecting a greater degree of influence from Western preoccupations with personal and emotional authenticity. Indeed, ongoing and consistent demonstrations of sentiment are necessary to ascertain another person's true moral character. Thuận underscored this with a Sino-Vietnamese proverb: *Họa hổ, họa bì, nan họa cốt. Tri nhân, tri diện, bất tri tâm* (Draw the tiger, draw its skin, but not its bones. Know the person, know the face, but not the heart).

IDENTIFYING *TÌNH CẢM*

As I was flipping through a paperback at a Phương Nam bookstore, a man in his twenties, eager to practice English with a foreigner, wondered aloud why I would be interested in a book entitled *The Sentimental Way of Life of the Vietnamese* (*Lối sống Tình cảm của Người Việt Nam*). He himself was holding a book on accounting principles. Before I could finish telling him that I was a graduate student researcher, he said, "I know now. You want to understand Vietnamese culture." Sentiment is a core concept that structures multiple identities in Vietnam, and people invoked it to me as perhaps the most fundamental component of Vietnamese society. For example, after the introduction, *The Sentimental Way* begins with a detailed description of funerary practices for one's parents, especially a father, to highlight such a funeral's status as the ultimate expression of both sentiment and cultural tradition. While these sweeping pronouncements should not be taken at face value, they do illuminate how people reflect on themselves by comparing themselves to an imagined Other. Here, I examine these often essentialist tropes to explore how ideas about sentiment are used to negotiate Ho Chi Minh City's increasingly diverse landscape of social identities.

According to a common adage, Vietnam is "a poor country but rich in spirit" (*nước nghèo, giàu tình cảm*). With a mix of pride and some embarrassment, people usually said it when offering me food or drink in their homes, as if to simultaneously highlight their generosity and apologize that they could not be more generous. The negative correlation between wealth and sentiment juxtaposes several tensions—between tradition and modernity, spirituality and materialism, and Vietnam and the West—that are crucial to many Ho Chi Minh City residents' sense of national and regional identity. Perhaps most important to this identity is the dichotomy between individuality and collectivism. For example, in Bác Lan's comparison of Vietnamese and Western mentalities, the latter are exoticized as wholly individualistic and independent.[3] Conversely, Bác Lan and many of her peers understand themselves, with a significant amount of ambivalence, to be collectively oriented and interdependent. Many argue that sentiment has the most important role in society because it provides the moral and emotional motivation for people to live cooperatively in the first place, and that members of societies with low levels of sentiment are prone to loneliness (*cô độc*). Again, this is an exaggeration of both Vietnam and the West and should not be accepted uncritically, but it does reveal key stakes around which identity is constructed.

Although at times my interlocutors spoke of it as emblematic of Vietnamese national culture, sentiment varies significantly throughout the country. The greatest distinction is made between rural and urban expressions of sentiment. Discourses of the nation portray cosmopolitan, urban, and modern Ho Chi Minh City as less Vietnamese than the traditional countryside or even than the much older and more "cultured" cities of Hanoi and Huế (cf. Harms 2011). For example, when I told Ho Chi Minh City residents (including my research assistant) that I was interested in discussing sentiment with them, they often suggested I conduct research in the heartland of the Mekong Delta instead. Khuyên, a nineteen-year-old woman, misses her hometown of Bến Tre, where people still have sentiment "without a shore" (*vô bờ*, meaning oceanic). A recent transplant to Ho Chi Minh City, she distrusts her new neighbors and disapproves of their conduct. According to her, when a person's desires are too easily met, as is the case in "modern" cities, then sentiment suffers because support and encouragement from others is no longer needed. Considering the dichotomy between tradition and modernity, some Ho Chi Minh City residents portrayed sentiment as an impediment to Vietnam's economic ambitions. For example, corrupt business practices were attributed not just to individual greed but also to the triumph of affective ties between partners over transparency and contractual negotiations.

Furthermore, variations in sentiment are used to demarcate regional differences. If social structure and family organization vary widely, then sentiment manifests differently from locale to locale because it is rooted in the specificities of various relationships. These regional distinctions are most marked in descriptions of northern and southern Vietnam. With its stronger Chinese influence, which Ho Chi Minh City residents often disparaged, the North features a rigid and elaborate patrilineal kinship system stemming from Confucianism. Conversely, the South has a more flexibly defined kinship system, a reflection of the cognatic kinship systems typically found in Southeast Asia (Luong 1984, 1989). Thus, the sentimental bonds between southerners are portrayed by both northerners and southerners as more fluid and ephemeral but genuine, while the bonds between northerners is considered more formal and permanent but forced.[4]

Regardless of these regional differences, people held up sentiment as the best of Vietnamese traditions. However, they have also become ambivalent toward these traditions. Sentiment and other supposed remnants of traditional culture are problematic for Ho Chi Minh City's middle class because they conflict with the modern lifestyles and individualized pursuit of wealth that have become emblematic of the reform era. For example, Vân-Anh, thirty-two, and I were on our way to pay our respects to a mutual friend's family after her father died. As our taxi climbed over a newly constructed bridge, Vân-Anh clucked in disapproval. "People used to help

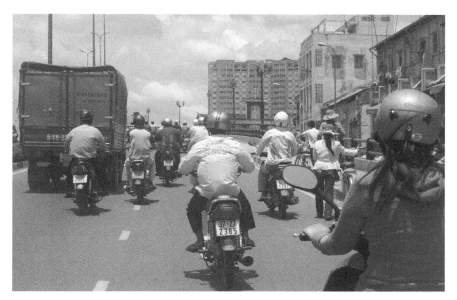

FIGURE 2. New infrastructure projects like the Ông Lãnh Bridge in District 4 ease congestion but also highlight inequality.

each other," she said. Looking out her window at a woman in her fifties pushing a food cart up the bridge's incline as motorbikes glided past her, she claimed that during the lean years of the postwar era a crowd of onlookers would have pushed the cart on the woman's behalf. People used to be always willing to help strangers, even when they had so little. Now that they could finally afford to be generous, they were unwilling to share. Our taxi driver chimed in to agree, citing numerous examples of a culture of self-interest that he saw every day from the driver's seat, as the car reached the other side of the bridge.

WORRIERS AND WARRIORS

When, during my fieldwork, people learned that I was from the United States, their questions usually focused on the details of everyday life in a country so many of them had fantasized about living in. How much are monthly electricity, water, and telephone bills? Is it true that you can get by with speaking only Vietnamese in the various Little Saigons? Does it snow in California? The answers to these questions helped them understand the lives of their relatives who had emigrated as refugees, and sometimes helped them imagine for themselves a life apparently free of worry. Hoa, however, had a different kind of question when we first met. "I heard that America has a lot of racism," she said. "Is it true?" Perhaps because moving to the United States was not as remote a possibility for Hoa as it had been, she wanted to assess possible threats. However, her question may have stemmed from something that was present in her life even before her sister got married. Hoa was a worrier. According to her, she had a pessimistic outlook on life and agonized over every decision she made, no matter how trivial. Even her father, who spent two years in a reeducation camp after the war, told her that she need not always assume that the worst would happen. Hoa often said that if she could change one thing about herself, it would be her insecurity and lack of confidence in her own abilities. Despite what she thinks about herself, her anxieties do not just reflect a nervous disposition. Rather, they are also rooted in family and gender expectations of sentiment and care.

Anthropological theories of care focus on the social relations that sustain life in states of emergency and banal normality alike, as well as considering how those relationships are implicated in political-economic forces (Buch 2015; Black 2018). That is, care is both a resource and a relational practice. While it includes a wide range of practices, here I focus on care as both a moral experience and a social obligation. Doing so focuses the analysis on the intersections of embodied experience, everyday practice, intergenerational relations, and political economy. Comparative analysis of caregiving is situated at the intersection of broad social transformations and intimate, everyday life. By considering the realities of care, including its stakes and barriers, anthropologists can examine the resources and practices that enable different kinds of people to live a meaningful life (Aulino 2019). As a social practice, care is contingent on who cares for whom and on the institutional and national policies that shape those roles. Care not only impacts those who receive it directly, but circulates across generations and communities.

Care can be translated in Vietnamese as nuôi (to nurture), chăm sóc (to look after or take care of), or quan tâm (to consider or be concerned with; lit., important to the heart). The most commonly discussed notion of care, quan tâm is evidence of sentimental attachment. To consider another is to assume their perspective and thereby anticipate their needs and wishes. Indeed, I found most Ho Chi Minh City residents to be close observers of others' behaviors—sometimes to the detriment, it seemed, of attending to their own feelings (see chapter 5). For example, as restaurant servers brought out the seafood dishes that Tuyết, forty-seven, had ordered for the table, she got up from her seat to direct their proper placement so that each guest would have easy access. Although the party of ten consisted mostly of her and her husband's friends, she hovered over her son and two of his friends (including me) to explain to us in detail what each dish was and which sauces to dip them in, point out the condiments on the table, and performatively ask me if I knew how to use chopsticks. I was getting hungry, and annoyed, so I quietly asked my friend why his mother was fussing so much. He pointedly responded, "Because she cares (quan tâm) about you." This form of care entails a thoughtful consideration of another person's desires and abilities while presuming the person's dependence and vulnerability. That is, it establishes a relationship based on caring and being cared for. Similarly, when Giang insisted on giving Hoa more spending money that she did not need, she reestablished a parent-child dynamic that perhaps had changed over the prior five years. Although Hoa still lived with her older sister, she had graduated from college and become engaged, markers of a burgeoning adulthood and independence. Hoa found the offer sweet, but I wonder if she ever chafed at her mother's good intentions.

In Vietnam, care is deeply intertwined with neo-Confucian hierarchical family structures and tied to an ethic of sacrifice, of submitting oneself to others, especially family members (Rydstrøm 2003a). The hierarchical nature of social relationships, often based on age and gender, is founded in what Shohet (2021) terms an *asymmetrical reciprocity* that fosters people's mutual caring and worrying. Epitomized by the aphorism *kính trên nhường dưới* (respect those above and yield to those below), asymmetrical reciprocity is first learned within the family, where filial piety (*hiếu thảo*) emphasizes respect for and subordination to one's elders, along with requisite support for one's juniors (Shohet 2013). Social roles for family members are strictly defined by gender. As the "pillar of the family" (*trụ cột gia đình*), fathers are responsible for the public face of the household, such as earning an income and participating in community organizations and rituals. Conversely, mothers' duties entail supporting and nurturing both their natal and their husband's families through domestic activities. Most relevant to Hoa, children are expected to obey their parents and, as they mature, fulfill a range of obligations related to care (Bayly 2020). For example, Khuyên's mother thinks that her daughter is mature for her age because she "never make[s] her sad" by going against her wishes. Within the family, harmony, rather than personal satisfaction, is the key measure of the ideal form of happiness (*hạnh phúc*; Taylor 1983; Kelley 2006; Pettus 2003). This kind of happiness is achieved when everyone carries out their assigned social roles and obligations, but it comes at a cost that is higher for some than for others.

According to many Ho Chi Minh City residents, in theory anybody has the potential to worry, but women consistently worry more than men. Despite the large number of historical and contemporary depictions of Vietnamese women as valiant warriors and "generals of the interior" (*nội tướng*; Tai 2001), most concur that women's social vulnerabilities make them more prone than men to worry about the future.[5] Furthermore, many of my interlocutors, including women, argued that women are more cautious, detail oriented, and emotionally sensitive than men. These supposed gender differences have become essentialized as a matter of instinct and subsequently naturalize sentiment and specific forms of worry and care as a preeminently feminine trait (Rydstrøm 2003b). Thus, the moral economy of care that sustains social ties depends on the greater social pressure for women to worry about others. That women in general—and mothers in particular—bear the burden of worrying is supported by a pervasive ethic of sacrifice (Tai 2001; Leshkowich 2006). For example, surrendering one's own time, energy, and physical and mental resources configures selfhood as morally upright. Furthermore, this devotional sacrifice should be performed without drawing attention to it; to be considered virtuous, one should bear suffering with acceptance and fortitude (Shohet 2021). Even taken as an essential quality of womanhood in and around Hanoi (Gammeltoft 2021), endurance (*chịu đựng*) is a testament not only to one's personal mettle but also to the strength of one's attachment to others. Open confrontations are typically avoided, especially if they would complicate implicit tensions within a family. For example, many of my interlocutors complained about their in-laws to me, but they would not voice those complaints to their spouses, because doing so would create more conflicts than resolutions. Even much of their own friends' advice is geared toward how to yield one's own happiness for the sake of the greater good, rather than helping them achieve their own goals.

However much Hoa hated them, her anxious traits were tied to what she valued most about herself: her pride in being a good daughter. She spoke rapturously about how much she loved her mother and worried constantly about her father, who suffered severe arthritis due to his treatment in the camps. She was their third child, so, under Vietnam's two-child policy, they were pressured by local officials to terminate the pregnancy and were penalized for refusing. Hoa would find moments throughout the day to perform small acts of care, such as making fresh orange juice during their lunchtime nap, not because it was requested or because she sought praise from them. Rather, she felt indebted to them for the sacrifices they had made just to give birth to her. For Hoa, worrying, when directed toward others, is enacted through distinct social relationships and inextricable from social institutions. Registering as a gendered form of care in Vietnam, worry is both a practice and a feeling state that transforms individuals into moral persons through a specific orientation to the needs of others. Anticipating the needs of others, especially one's family and neighbors, is both a moral duty and an economic strategy (Dao 2020). While overtly worrying for someone in a vulnerable position in the United States implies that the object of worry is not self-sufficient, doing so in Vietnam is acceptable, since people readily acknowledge their dependence on others. Indeed, pity, compassion, and affection are closely linked, and people under duress may seek out the pity of others as affirmation of their circumstances.

MORAL BREAKDOWNS

That afternoon when Hoa told me of her apprehensions over her imminent move to the United States, I asked her what she was most worried about. She could not pick a single thing because she was anxious about everything—even not knowing what to be anxious about. Hoa knew that her entire life was about to be transformed, but she did not know what it would be transformed into. On the verge of what felt like being cut off from the relationships that were fundamental to her sense of self, Hoa found herself unmoored, and in this crisis of meaning the rest of her world followed suit. Anxiety corrupts and undermines the meanings of bedrock assumptions about the world, as well as the very means of making meaning (Kristeva 1982; Salecl 2004). That is, anxiety in its most potent states is not just meaningless—it also makes everything around it so. Hoa was the envy of her peers, many of whom dreamed of studying abroad, especially in the United States, and the pressure to put on a happy face prevented her from sharing her troubles with most of them. Her worrying-about, focused on her own unknown fate, cast her as selfish and ungrateful. Her emotional breakdown was becoming a moral one too.

In our conversations about morality (*đạo đức*), Ho Chi Minh City residents often offered a simple phrase to sum it up: "It's complicated (*phức tập*)." Many stated that such complications made it difficult to discuss moral behavior. In a possible attempt to avoid the topic entirely, Phong, a thirty-one-year-old man, offered to buy me a fifth-grade civics reader, where I could learn to follow the ultimate role model of Ho Chi Minh himself by dressing simply and humbly and loving the nation as one's family. Proper morality is communicated in state media and schools, where a moral education is considered just as important as a scientific and literary one (Bayly 2020). Moreover, Confucian principles also specify moral codes of behavior. For example, the "three obediences and four virtues" (*tam tòng tứ đức*) prescribe that women are to obey their fathers, husbands, and sons (after their husbands die) and comport themselves with modesty in speech, manners, and work. Proper morality in Vietnam is typically framed in terms of absolute virtues such as patriotism and filial piety. While the standards of being an obedient child or upstanding citizen may be relatively clear, however, living up to them can still be difficult for the individuals who occupy those roles, especially when they do not make sense anymore. Perhaps this is why Phong was so uninterested in the topic.

How people navigate shifting ethical terrain provides insight into the construction of moral behavior and personhood. Anthropological scholarship has moved beyond analyzing static doctrines explicitly delineated as moral to differentiate normative social values from moral and ethical quandaries (Laidlaw 2002; Robbins 2013). Moral behavior cannot be reduced to a set of absolute principles or prescriptive principles found in sacred texts, and people are not moral just because they comply with conventional regulations. In other words, the moral and the social cannot be reduced to each other. Instead, people may strive toward an ethics that is fragmented, ambivalent, and contingent upon the situations that they find themselves in. Zigon (2010) proposes such moral breakdowns to be productive for ethnographic analyses of morality because they disrupt the relation between paradigmatic social norms and everyday experiences of morality. In these instances, people are forced to negotiate conflicting demands to achieve moral selfhood. Indeed, a relational ethics is grounded in care and concern for the space between people (Zigon 2021). Moral breakdowns are a problematization of everyday moral dispositions and provide people with an opportunity to reflect on everyday, taken-for-granted ideals of morality and instead "work on themselves and, in so doing, alter their very way of being-in-the-world" (Zigon 2007, 138). However, anthropological theorizing on moralities has largely ignored the question of how emotions and sentiments are invoked in this moral reasoning, as well as their implications for organizing human sociality (Throop 2012).

Throughout Vietnam, people tend to be drawn to moral ambiguities more than to absolute principles (Shohet 2021). The lists of proper behaviors according to socialist morality (e.g., dressing humbly and following Ho Chi Minh as a role model) that they memorized in school are of little use in determining what makes a good (*tốt bụng*, kindhearted, lit. good stomach) person in ethically ambiguous contexts. Rather, moral reasoning is guided, to a great extent, by sentimental ties.[6] A paragon of moral virtue is someone who is "blinded by sentiment" (*quảng mù tình cảm*) to the point of sacrificing their financial and emotional resources and even compromising their own virtue to someone who does not deserve such devotion.[7] People living according to sentiment (*căn cớ tình cảm*) may well realize that they are being manipulated (*lôi kéo*), but seem powerless to advocate for themselves. These situations become particularly difficult when sentiment, romantic love, and platonic affection/compassion/pity are intertwined. For example, when Khuyên was eight months old, her father abandoned her and her mother to move to the United States with his first wife. Her mother's relatives told her he was untrustworthy during their courtship, but she continued the relationship regardless. Furthermore, Khuyên, who knows the pain he inflicted on her mother and long resented him for it, told me she does not want to hate him anymore. Instead, she feels oddly proud of his accomplishments, from what little she knows of him (e.g., he is a hospital administrator). Both Khuyên and her mother demonstrate sentiment that requires significant forgiveness. Supporting loved ones, even when they are in the wrong, often takes precedence over a commitment to moral principle. Ethical behavior is more a matter of a practiced heart or a finely tuned instinct than of strict adherence to rules and decorum (Gammeltoft 2018). It stems from being keenly attuned to others as fellow moral selves so that one is able to anticipate and meet their needs and share in life's ups and downs (Marr 2000). Thus, although morality in Vietnam is guided by normative expectations of one's own behavior, a person's moral character emerges through social relationships.

Sentiment is a critical component in the assemblage of discourses and practices that are broadly constructed as morality (Zigon 2010). Bayly (2020) argues that the "essence of moral agency" in Vietnam lies in a "warmth of feeling conveyed aloud as a bond of care and conscience" (37). Thus, care is not just required for sociality to function but is also a matter of morality. For example, Thiên, a seventy-year-old man, told me that "people with sentiment are different than those without. If I don't have any feelings about a friend, then it doesn't create any sentiment. If you want to have sentiment, then you have to have love (*tình thương*), and vice versa."

According to him, an insensitive (*vô cảm*) person would be someone who feels nothing upon seeing a baby. Lacking an instant connection and a heart, their emotions are "brittle (*khô cứng*) with regard to collectives (*tập thể*) and communities (*cộng đồng*)." Moral actions must be motivated by one's own genuine concern for others. Conversely, the same actions, when mandated by decree or formality, are considered mechanical. For Thiên, "the heart decides everything." Personhood and morality are inextricable: smooth, nonconfrontational sociality depends on constant attention, accommodation, and adjustment to others, and everyday moral actions are concerned with one's indeterminate and fluid orientation toward care for others.

When Hoa told her mother of her misgivings, Giang replied that her sister needed her help. In fact, the entire family needed her. Now that her parents were retired, Hoa was to be the family's primary breadwinner by becoming a pharmacist in the United States and sending economic remittances to Vietnam. (Her older brother seemed unable or uninterested in providing for his natal family, and Hoa rarely mentioned him in our conversations.) Thus, the money that Hoa's parents borrowed from relatives and banks alike was an investment in the future for a family that had long lived on the edges of poverty. At a disadvantage due to their unfavorable political history, they struggled more than most to make ends meet after the war, yet they were able to pay for their children's education. Despite her upward mobility, Hoa felt she had less in common with her classmates at university than with her friends and relatives in Đồng Nai Province. This devotion to family was used to help motivate her to leave but also made the prospect that much harder for her.

This cultural model of worry articulates it as a moral experience by providing a framework within which anxiety is made meaningful as a reflection of one's devotion, care, and sacrifice to others. The (negatively valued) existential suffering of *worrying about something* becomes a moral sentiment when it is understood as *worrying about someone*. That is, emotional relations to others, vis-à-vis notions of care and consideration (*quan tâm*), are forged by worrying-for. Here, experiencing "concern for an Other, which grows into some sense that one wants to make their lives possible," is the basis for moral experience (Parish 2014, 34). Sentiment renders moral behavior subjectively meaningful, as Bác Dũng, a sixty-six-year-old man, describes: "People with *tình cảm* are different than those without. If I don't have any feelings about a friend then it doesn't create any sentiment. If you have sentiment, you have to love, and vice versa. The heart of a person who sees something like a baby . . . and doesn't know how to love it is numb. . . . Their feelings are brittle."

When discussing issues of morality, Ho Chi Minh City residents often invoke suffering, for the truest test and indication of people's morality emerges from their suffering. Notions of morality are crucial in articulating suffering in meaningful terms (Das et al. 2000). Vietnam's "valorization of suffering" (Jellema 2005) and "cult of melancholy" (Nash and Nguyen 1995) play an integral role in the construction of moral personhood. Kate Jellema (2005) argues that revolutionary and socialist politics reoriented merit toward suffering for the nation. While in domestic arenas it typically refers to yielding one's own interests (Shohet 2021), *sacrifice* (*hy sinh*) in state discourse refers to soldiers dying on the battlefield or to mothers whose sons became martyrs (*liệt sĩ*) to the revolution (Kwon 2008; McElwee 2005; Tai 2001). For Buddhists, merit (*công*) is acquired by performing good deeds without an expectation of reciprocity (Jellema 2005). These means of finding meaning in suffering provide a model for how worrying-about is transformed into worrying-for.

In spite of the attempts to keep her uncertainties unsaid, Hoa got into an argument with her sister over the phone and told her that she did not want to live with her anymore, before breaking into tears. Indeed, she broke into tears upon recounting this to me, pained not just by her own misfortune but also by the hurt she had caused her sister with her admission. Many young people in Ho Chi Minh City, including Hoa, describe remaining silent (*im lặng*) as one of the best tools at their disposal to subdue their tempers and prevent moral transgressions, especially disrespect to their elders. For them, controlling one's emotions is principally about their expression, not modifying their inner experience. (However, this pattern has been changing in recent years, as will be discussed in chapter 5.) Although Hoa did not consider her doubts about her future plans to be immoral per se, she found it difficult to reconcile her personal anxieties with the love and filial devotion she felt—or wanted to feel—toward her family. To her, these anxieties were evidence of the insecure nature that she disliked about herself, as well as a sign of insufficient trust in and gratitude for her family's plans. This moral breakdown led to an opportunity for self-reflection for Hoa and perhaps played a role in her eventual self-transformation.

Staying in Vietnam would allow Hoa to maintain the role of a daughter, yet would also be a failure to live up to that role.[8] Backing out of the plans now would be both a personal and a family failing. To her, the constant worrying over matters, trivial and otherwise, was evidence of her insecure nature—what she often said she hated most about herself and hoped to overcome as she gained confidence with age. The more positive evaluation of worrying-for than of worrying-about creates a form of moral personhood that casts Hoa's anxieties in a negative light. Perhaps it is at this intersection of conflicting ideas, feelings, and desires that Hoa might come to terms not just with moral discourses and sentiments, but with the ethical dilemma she found herself in. But questioning her relationship with her family and their designs for her seemed to be too painful, too anxiety-inducing to endure.

Ultimately, Hoa succeeded not through renegotiating the standards placed on her but through abiding by them. She was motivated to worry-for not because it was something she necessarily wanted to do but because it made her who she wanted to be. The intentional act of worrying-for is part of being a good person, yet despite the explicit attempts to socialize and cultivate anxiety as a moral sentiment, it is also understood by many of my interlocutors as an innate reaction for someone who has the capacity to worry (i.e., someone who cares for others). Her anxiety was experienced as a "relational intertwining" as she attuned her own sensibilities to the needs of her family (Zigon 2021, 388). Anxiety produces moral personhood when it is transformed from a subjectively devalued feeling to an intersubjectively valorized sentiment. As Hoa discovered, this process is often tenuous and does not ensure success.

CONCLUSION

How people worry for each other reveals their commitments to and entanglements in the world. Instead of assuming the distinctions between subject and object, focusing on worry as a moral sentiment highlights how those distinctions are made, felt, and registered at bodily and communal levels (Mattingly and Throop 2018). From a perspective on anxiety that frames it as a social practice rather than an individual possession, extreme worry is a normal, even necessary part of everyday life, rather than an exceptional state of pathology. The Vietnamese moral economy of anxiety reveals how worry—simultaneously thought, affect, and practice—generates and sustains selfhood. In contrast to a Western conception of anxiety as an indication of the individual's worth on account of their own business, industriousness, and importance, the cultural model of anxiety in Vietnam frames care and sacrifice as indication of an individual's moral sentiment enacted in the service of others. However, the construction of moral personhood is an uncertain process that cannot be reduced to individual projects of self-making or to the ideals imposed on them by others (Pandian 2009). Rather, breakdowns and fault lines in these ideals can be just as productive to moral reasoning.

Seen in the context of care, sacrifice, and gender, the models and instances of worry that my participants spoke of were framed as distinctively Vietnamese. Worry, I was often told, came naturally to them because of a long history of collective and individual hardship. However, as the country's economic future brightens, some Ho Chi Minh City residents worry about the state of worrying-for. Several years after Vân-Anh lamented the decline of moral sentiments to me in a taxi, I paid her and her mother, Hương, a visit as part of the Tết (Lunar New Year) festivities. During Tết, most of Ho Chi Minh City's restaurants and markets are closed. Fearing that I would go hungry, Hương began to fill a large shopping bag for me with fruit and a container of fried rice that she had cooked in anticipation of stores closing, despite my repeated insistence that I had adequately prepared for the holidays. Out of the corner of my eye, I could see Vân-Anh laughing at my failure to convince her mother otherwise. She later told me she was amused not just because she could tell that I did not want to take the food but also because she knew that she used to be like her mother. "But these days I'm too busy with work," she said. "I have to live for myself" (*sống cho mình*). The next chapter examines the implications of Vân-Anh's apparent change of heart. To what extent is her fatalism toward worry as a moral sentiment warranted? What are the effects of the decreased viability of a model of worrying-for on the experience of anxiety? What, if anything, has emerged in its wake?

3

Rich Sentiments

Sometime in the late 1990s, "emotion" (*cảm xúc*) became trendy in Vietnam. Its popularity, I was told, began after one of the first extended broadcasts of a foreign television series in the country, a South Korean soap opera whose title, *Neukkim* (*Feelings*), was translated as *Cảm Xúc*. The word *cảm xúc*, which once had a primarily academic connotation, appears in advertisements for tour packages to Singapore. The brand name of my friend's Thai-manufactured Honda motorbike knockoff is "Feelings."[1] Customers at the Maximark supermarket food court can order a *cảm xúc* coffee, a standard Vietnamese iced milk coffee but with additional cherry syrup. The opening of the lush Café Cảm Xúc in the city's former French quarter was followed by a number of imitation "emotion cafés." Unlike the informal sidewalk cafés[2] with their tightly packed rows of chairs facing the mayhem of Ho Chi Minh City's traffic, the inward spatial arrangement of these cafés, with customers seated in front of each other across a small table, facilitates a face-to-face emotional exchange between customers. The primary allure of the emotion cafés is not the quality or uniqueness of the drinks—most of their menus are identical—but rather the wide spaces and spectacles of waterfalls, light displays, and koi fish ponds. The emotions of these emotion cafés are to be experienced and displayed in the open alongside the crowds of fellow patrons who rove from café to café in search of the next most fashionable nightspot. Today, the emotion cafés sit largely empty as customers increasingly prefer smaller venues tucked away in the cramped city center's alleys. The seating is set up to enclose spaces that foster intimacy with one's companions instead of a celebration of consumption in open areas. The interior design elements are less opulent and emphasize details over spectacle to encourage the use of close-up, high-resolution photography. Pictures geotagged from these locations on Instagram often feature people with wistful expressions, staring off into the distance or reading a book. The affects displayed at these cafés are directed not just toward a person's companions but to an audience mediated by phones, reflecting the evolution of the aesthetic appreciation of subjective states

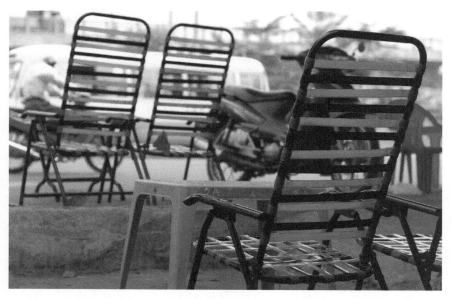

FIGURE 3. A sidewalk café in Bình Thạnh District faces customers toward the street instead of each other.

among the middle class. These commercial fads were tentative when I first noticed them in 2007, but they foreshadowed a remarkable advancement of the emotions in Ho Chi Minh City's public spaces.

Of course, various discourses and expressions that are broadly emotional in nature have long been prominent in Vietnamese social life (Jamieson 1995). While *cảm xúc* is the Vietnamese word that best conveys the meaning of emotion as it is understood in English, it is not the most commonly used one. Rather, *sentiment (tình cảm)* occupies much of the same semantic space as *emotion* does in English, in addition to denoting people's feelings for others. Thus, it describes the emotional connections between people rather than an individual's state of feeling. In contrast to Ho Chi Minh City residents' associations between sentiment and Vietnamese tradition, the new and sometimes contradictory meanings attached to *cảm xúc* signify the socioeconomic changes of the reform era. The rapid emergence of *cảm xúc* as a seemingly new addition to contemporary life is not limited to market goods.[3] The commodities attached to *cảm xúc* do not promise to induce a specific feeling such as joy or excitement. Rather, their allure stems from shifting perceptions of emotion (or perhaps of being emotional) itself. Increased financial resources may certainly be understood to allow people to explicitly dwell upon their feelings instead of attending solely to basic survival, but they are not wholly sufficient to account for the particular forms that emotion has taken in Vietnam.

Rather, the reconceptualization of self and society in an affective register is not merely the result of Vietnam's version of neoliberalism but instead is critical to

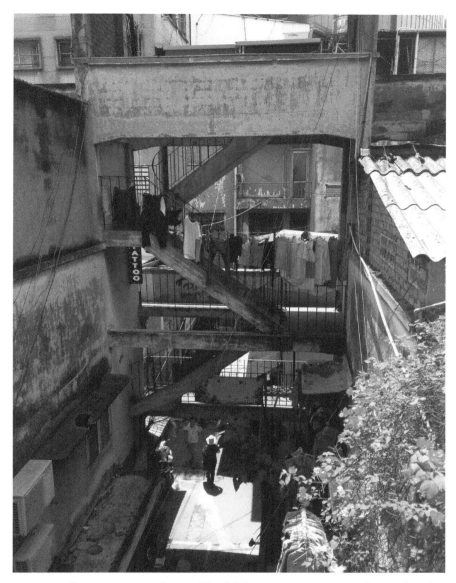

FIGURE 4. The apartment complex at 14 Tôn Thất Đạm Street in District 1 is the site of trendy cafés, vintage clothing stores, and private residences.

the process of neoliberalization itself. What social conditions make feelings worth categorizing? How are new understandings of emotion used to reimagine one's self and its place in the world? What is the relationship between emotion as a social construct and emotion as a self process? Within popular discourses of modernity, the rising middle class's culture of self-interest threatens the Confucian and socialist ethics of collective sacrifice and restraint exemplified by notions of *tình cảm* (Shohet 2013; King et al. 2008).[4] However, it can also be understood as emerging alongside and in response to Confucian and socialist principles. In identifying and categorizing various feelings, including anxiety, as explicitly "emotional" in nature, people participate in a self-fashioning project that cultivates an inner self that, while informed by neoliberal sensibilities, does not wholly replace socialist or Confucian models of selfhood.

While forms of largely middle-class selfhood in Vietnam are increasingly thematized as "emotional," it would be a mistake to assume an automatic correlation with intensely felt affective experiences. Rather than implying that the emotional lives of lower-class Ho Chi Minh City residents or people living before 1986 are simpler or shallower than those of people today, the growing popularity of *cảm xúc* suggests that people are rethinking the significance of emotion in their personal and social lives. Although ideas about and experiences of emotion should not be conflated, neither should they be dichotomized. Furthermore, people do not simply feel "emotion." Rather, they feel specific affective experiences that they may have learned to identify with the general category of emotion. Indeed, this process is what many Ho Chi Minh City residents are increasingly taking for granted, in turn naturalizing not only *cảm xúc* but also the political-economic regimes that have made the new social forms associated with it possible. In order to avoid reproducing Western conceptualizations of emotion, I examine a changing ethnopsychology of how emotions arise and are interpreted and experienced (Lutz 1988) and analyze how it becomes internalized by Ho Chi Minh City residents. Their folk models of emotion, sentiment, and selfhood at times contradict and coincide with each other's, revealing the emergence of the new meanings that emotion takes on.

RETURNED SPIRITS

In general, the entire spirit of ancient times . . . and the present time . . . may be summed up in two words: "I" and "we". . . . Our lives now lie within the sphere of "I." Having lost breadth, we seek depth. But the deeper we go, the colder it gets. . . . Along with our sense of superiority, we have lost even the peace of mind of previous times. . . . The West has returned our spirit to us.
—HOÀI THANH (1988 [1942], QUOTED IN NINH 2002, 24)

Hoài Thanh, a literary critic writing in the 1930s and '40s, underscored many of the same doubts about the self that still haunt Vietnamese today. Anticolonial reformers at the beginning of the twentieth century blamed the failure of Vietnamese resistance to French conquest in the late 1800s on the inadequacy of Confucian principles to withstand incursion from the West. Subsequent debates about societal reform often centered on the extent to which Confucian norms or French notions of civilization should shape the "inner spirit" of the Vietnamese or the outer or secondary aspects of modern Vietnamese society (Ninh 2002). By the 1920s, alternative discourses of civilization were appropriated to reconsider individual behavior and obligations toward society. Neologisms for the individual (*cá nhân*), society (*xã hội*), and democracy (*dân chủ*), among others, further engaged with Western forms of modernity that took a self-reflexive turn to relationships between the individual and state (Marr 2000; Taylor 1989; Giddens 1991; Beck 1992).

Its supporters considered the eventual spread of socialism throughout Vietnam a dramatic break with past ways of relating to one another as well as to oneself. Institutions and ideologies associated with anything considered feudal or foreign were demonized as antithetical to the goal of a new socialist modernity (Tai 1992; Taylor 2001). In order to redirect people's primary obligations from filial ties to the nation, the state emphasized affectively laden ideologies of utopianism, egalitarianism, and patriotic sacrifice. Christina Schwenkel's (2013) concept of "socialist affect" traces the affective mobilization of social and political action in northern Vietnam and how it shaped, and still resonates with, present subjectivities and the everyday experience of capitalism. The Communist Party promised a future of prosperity achievable through collectivist projects that engineered both urban infrastructure and workers' profound attachments to socialist ideals, to each other, and to the ends and means of labor itself. State discourses were designed to counter dwindling morale with utopian sentiments. However, when such promises never materialized, the objects of these affections came to represent both the state's inability to care for its citizens and their own exclusion from the radical change of course that the state subsequently pursued with *đổi mới*. The fate of the "individual" in Vietnam's discourse of society has gone from the denigration of selfishness during the various stages of collectivizing reforms starting in 1954 in the (northern) Democratic Republic of Vietnam and in 1975 in the (southern) Republic of Vietnam to the post-reform celebration of individual ingenuity (MacLean 2008).

As average incomes throughout Vietnam rise, a consumerist pursuit of cultivating one's own identity has taken precedence over sacrificing for the nation. After years of isolation from much of the world, many in Ho Chi Minh City have access to a global culture of consumerism and self-interest that would have been difficult to fathom a generation ago. Once criticized for its associations with selfishness under collectivist policies, the "individual" is now celebrated within Vietnam's discourse of society for its ingenuity and adaptability in a market economy (MacLean 2008). Although colonialism, socialism, and neoliberalism have all focused on establishing a Vietnamese form of modernity (Brook and Luong 1997; Leshkowich 2006; Marr 2003; McHale 2004; Turley 1993), it is primarily projects associated with the colonial and neoliberal eras that have legitimized individualism, often through individualized consumption, as a means to become a new type of Vietnamese citizen (Vann 2012).

Rather than marking a simple transition from socialism to neoliberalism, recent changes in self-understanding demonstrate the reaches of both political-economic regimes and reveal that no steady teleology runs through Confucianism, colonialism, socialism, and neoliberalism. Thus, like so many other neoliberal projects throughout the region, the very incompleteness of *đổi mới* suggests that neoliberalism is best viewed, not as a monolithic and autonomous entity, but as a historically contingent set of divergent practices and institutions that encourage or stem from the deregulation of economic activity and the privatization of formerly public domains (Nguyễn-Võ 2008; Schwenkel and Leshkowich 2012).[5] Anthropological approaches to *đổi mới* retheorize neoliberalism from the perspective of everyday life as an alternative approach to totalizing master narratives about global conditions and highlight "the fluidity and coarticulation by which new subjectivities are being formed that are neither clearly socialist nor clearly neoliberal in their identity" (Pashigian 2012, 532).

SENTIMENT AND/OR EMOTION

Despite their overlap, the ways that *tình cảm* (sentiment, emotion) and *cảm xúc* (emotion, feelings) are conceptualized, monitored, and discussed have different implications for selfhood. Although the contrasts between sentiment and emotion can be subtle to the point where many of my interlocutors could scarcely differentiate them during interviews, they are being made more explicit by mostly younger and highly educated members of a growing middle and upper class in Ho Chi Minh City. An alternative discourse of the self, one based on *cảm xúc*, is being carved out of notions of *tình cảm* as many Ho Chi Minh City residents relate a wide range of emotional experiences to each other under the conceptual umbrella of *cảm xúc*. Increasingly influential Cartesian models of the self in which personal identity is located in the recesses of one's private thoughts certainly play a role in this shift (Lutz 1988; Dixon 2012). However, the Vietnamese theory of affective life is not merely becoming Westernized, and the role of *tình cảm* in the construction of the self is not just being supplanted by *cảm xúc*. Rather, the categorization of feeling is made possible through a redefinition and reorganization of the emotions that is being worked through preexisting understandings of sentiment.

Although *cảm xúc* more frequently refers to a broader range of subjective feeling states than *tình cảm*, it also connotes a similar meaning as *tình cảm*, in much the same way that *feelings* does in the English-language expression *to have feelings for someone* (i.e., to be romantically attracted to someone). If *tình cảm* principally refers to enduring bonds between people, then *cảm xúc* is considered a slighter and more capricious variant because of its associations with the initial stages of infatuation that have not yet become known and, therefore, made real to others through verbal expression. Thus, the attachments of *cảm xúc* are less durable, reliable, and trustworthy because its occurrence and experience are more interior.

Cảm xúc is alternately conceptualized as a subcategory of sentiment or a necessary step toward sentiment. From this perspective, there are no such things as "pure feelings"; rather, various feeling states are primarily considered vehicles for the evaluation of positions from which an individual is to make moral judgments.

Thus, for many in Vietnam, to conceptualize affective experience as a primarily abstract, interior, and mental state and as a classification of discrete feeling states such as anger, sadness, and boredom is a fairly new trend, since the distinction between one's affective bonds with other people and how one feels about anything else is not explicit. Many were aware of the dual meanings of *tình cảm* as both sentiment and emotion, but, in articulating their models of how it worked, rarely differentiated them. The construction of the emotions as a neutral, stand-alone category for our feelings is itself rooted in Western philosophy. Early nineteenth-century psychologists replaced theories of immoral passions and moral affections with a new conceptualization of the emotions as psychophysiological energies that are bodily and irrational, secular and morally disengaged, and uncontrollable and spontaneous (Dixon 2012).

However, the scientific disciplining of the emotions in Vietnam is not limited to the *đổi mới* era. In the prominent scholar Đào Duy Anh's *Sino-Vietnamese Dictionary* (1932), *cảm xúc* was defined by the *thất tình*, or seven emotions: *hỉ* (joy), *ái* (love), *nộ* (anger), *ố* (hatred), *lạc* (happiness), *bi* (pain), and *ai* (melancholy). Relating to a theory of excessive emotion as a pathogen,[6] this set stems from the *qiqing* (seven emotional reactions) of traditional Chinese medicine. However, currently the *thất tình* are not widely known in Vietnam to nonspecialists in Eastern medicine or philosophy.[7] A more contemporary definition of *cảm xúc* reflects the new criteria for the emotions: a vibration in the heart/gut through exposure to something (Viện Ngôn ngữ học 2002). In this definition, *cảm xúc* shifts from a delimited set of feeling states to a more abstract physiological principle that allows for the incorporation of a broader range of psychosocial experiences. Ironically, this produces a greater proliferation of categories that can be used to psychologize more elements of social life.

For example, Châu, a thirty-year-old international NGO worker who proudly describes herself as a "modern and sensitive woman," said, "If explained according to science, then the emotions are what enters your eyes, then has an effect in the brain, and then in your heart so there's some substance that pushes through the body and makes you have an emotion in your heart." Looking back on her twenties, she speculated that she had spent so much time in her room by herself to avoid any interactions that would inexplicably (even to her) leave her in tears. For her, a wide range of stimuli can turn into an emotion. The shift from sentiment as an ethical relationship to emotion as a physical substance took a metaphysical turn in a more romantic definition given by Vy, a college student, to her boyfriend Thuận at a party: *cảm xúc là khí trong lòng* (emotion is the energy in the gut/heart). This conceptualization repurposes the cosmological principle of *khí* (*qi* in Chinese) to reflect the Western theory of emotion as an internal substance. However, that it was mocked by her friends as maudlin reflects how *cảm xúc* is still couched in a discourse of romance. Models of emotion and selfhood shape the parameters of who people think they could be, who they want to be, and who they think they should be. Châu and Vy elaborate on the conceptual distinctions between *cảm xúc* and *tình cảm* not only to explain their respective introversion and romanticism, which were criticized as excessive by their families, but also to assert an emotive self that differs from models of selfhood rooted in sentiment. The emotive self is particularly appealing to them and to other mostly young, middle-class residents of Ho Chi Minh City because it orients them toward new opportunities and challenges of *đổi mới*–era Vietnam.

ACCOUNTS OF EMOTION

The contemporary transformations of affect, emotion, and the self in Vietnam can be further seen in the stories told through which human nature "discovers" itself. The current popularization of emotion is driven by the supposed scientific and medical expertise of sources such as advice columns and translations of Western self-help books that became available when Vietnam's isolationist period ended in 1986. Online message boards and social media (*mạng xã hội*) have recently become popular sources of information and misinformation about self-care and wellness strategies, psychiatric diagnoses, and mental health services. Although the formal study of academic psychology in Vietnam is limited largely to educational psychology, general interest in the field is pervasive, with avid readers hoping to unlock the secrets of human nature. Common assumptions that Western academic psychology has deepened people's understandings of the emotions (rather than shifting the terms of the conversation themselves) depict prior understandings of emotion as simplistic or incorrect. For example, despite his evident knowledge of and respect for Eastern philosophy, Thầy Vững, a seventy-year-old retired professor, posited that scientific advances had increased the amount of known emotions in Vietnam from seven to more than five hundred. Notions of the *thất tình* now appear even more antiquated when compared to contemporary psychological theories of the mind that posit a seemingly infinite combination of emotional experiences.

The advances of psychologically oriented discourses of the emotions not only make prior theories of emotion seem meager but minimize the impact of the social institutions that once supported them. Voicing common anxieties about people's evolving lifestyles, Mai, a forty-year-old entrepreneur, asserted that sentiment still plays an important role in her life but is fast becoming a relic of Vietnamese traditions that are increasingly at odds with the country's integration into the global economy: "The Vietnamese are actually a people that live mainly through sentiment, so people decide things based on sentiment alone. There aren't any principles. Principles are principles. If you satisfy me and my demands, then it's OK. . . . Westerners understand that you have to have principles in life and can't base everything on sentiment. Vietnam still isn't familiar with these principles because we've had this ideology that's been passed down from grandfather to father (*ý thức hệ từ đời ông đời cha*). It's in our genes now."

Hierarchical social relationships are often blamed for the previous dearth of attention to people's inner lives. Many in Vietnam have strong memories of their strict upbringing and heard stories of their own parents' even more severe childhoods. As a result of the unquestioned internalization of parents' perspectives, according to Mai's argument, people grow up alienated from their own needs and desires. Mai assumes an internal and perduring self that can exist, at least in a diminished form, apart from active cultivation and engagement with others, waiting to be discovered. The logic that people set aside either "traditional" beliefs to better understand their true nature and access their psychic potential naturalizes both forms of modernity and their transformation of affect.

Accounts that highlight the influence of modernization on recent changes in people's emotional lives focus on the diversity of choice in post-reform Vietnam. A wide array of choices now characterizes self-cultivation and the social identities that define the self. According to this explanation, with access to more choices and greater control over their lives, modern, enlightened people presumably had richer emotional lives that were untethered to "tradition." For example, Hoàng, a thirty-three-year-old psychiatrist, asked me in casual conversation where I found my "joy" (*niềm vui*). His choice of that word is notable in that he did not ask about "happiness" (*hạnh phúc*), which is traditionally defined by family cohesion and cooperativeness. Conversely, his definition of joy entails having an interesting job that earns enough money to pursue everyday pleasures. Hoàng emphasizes an individually cultivated sense of satisfaction that emerges from making self-motivated choices within a crowded marketplace of options. When considering a career change that would engage his interests more extensively, Hoàng himself found inspiration in what he saw as an emphasis on inner passion as a motivating force that was not as widely available before *đổi mới*.

Hoàng's question stands in contrast to a recent past when, according to many of my interlocutors, extreme suffering stunted people's souls as much as their bodies. Because the rise of emotion is often associated with self-discovery, pre-reform subjectivity was depicted by some as barren and emotionally bereft. People with few memories of the Vietnam-American War and its immediate aftermath imagined the process of understanding the self during those difficult circumstances to be found in the actions needed for basic survival, not direct self-contemplation. For example, a twenty-four-year-old self-styled polymath who gave herself the nickname "Vic" claimed that the definition of happiness was one of the main differences between her and her parents' and grandparents' generations. She parlayed her considerable marketing savvy into high-profile jobs that permitted extensive overseas travel. Meanwhile, her mother worried that Vic's outspokenness and wanderlust might cause people from her rural hometown to deem her ill-bred and unfit for marriage, at least to a "traditional" Vietnamese man. According to Vic, those who came of age under privation emphasize stability in their version of happiness. Parents want their children to be happy, but what makes both parents and children happy is not the same thing. Echoing Anh and Mai's conflicts with their parents, Vic's argument alludes to mutual understanding as a resolution to the unintended conflicts produced by her generation's emotional expectations. She deems prior means of self-discovery to be haphazard and contingent on external factors in order to be a genuine self-fashioning project, reflecting the increased psychologization of social life following đổi mới.

In the midst of the emotional awakening of the reform era, many people expressed anxieties about an accompanying emotional fallout. Linh, a forty-six-year-old counselor, echoed the widespread notion that people's emotional lives have deepened in recent years but, unlike Vic's more optimistic reading of emotional life in contemporary Vietnam, focuses on the dangers ahead: "Vietnam is on a path of development after years of famine, sickness, war, and scarcity. Then, people only worried about food and clothing; they only ate enough to feel full and wore enough to warm themselves. . . . Now things are modern and civilized. Material needs have limits, but spiritual needs are bigger. Nobody's cared about them until now. From here on out people will care more about them because as society develops people will confront spiritual crises." Common anxieties over the increasing soullessness of modern life and a supposedly unmoored sense of self link modernity with the waning of sentiment. According to this logic, the frenetic pace of life in contemporary Ho Chi Minh City that partly makes more proactive self-cultivation possible also threatens the intimate social bonds that have been used as a self-conscious marker of national identity (Trương 2009).

However, the material comforts and cultures of self-interest associated with modernity do not just allow for certain people to "get in touch with their feelings" as if they were waiting to be activated. A number of my respondents even suggested that before đổi mới, people experienced their feelings only superficially. However, when I asked them to reflect further on this claim, many of them reversed their positions. That this characterization is so widespread, yet does not stand up to much scrutiny, reflects the persistence of the imagined links between modernity, progress, and individual self-discovery. Rather, the various passions that were idealized or motivated for political ends during the country's colonial, war, or immediate postwar eras were certainly deeply felt by many people, but the new subjectivity—psychological, political, class, or otherwise—that is offered by đổi mới and the immense potential it offers are connected with different affective and material desires that have become central to what it currently means to be

Vietnamese. In blaming a history of feudal traditions, war, and poverty for people's detachment from their emotions, now so emblematic of human nature, Ho Chi Minh City residents render prior political regimes a violation of their humanity.

Popular notions of emotional life after 1986 assume that modernity offers people a way to combat a perceived alienation from their own individual selves. However, it is not just Confucian and socialist legacies that may have alienated people from their feelings. Perhaps just as culpable for the increased attention on this emotional fallout is the newfound emphasis on emotion, which is characterized as innate to human beings yet also somewhat foreign to Vietnamese culture. People are not merely "freed" from prior regimes of governance, but must be made free by instilling different notions of and relationships to social life (Rose 1999). The collective reckoning of sentiment's purported fall and emotion's rise assumes a modernist teleology and has compromised the long-standing sources of the social identities that inform selfhood as people turn inward.

THE RENOVATED SELF: NEOLIBERAL, SOCIALIST, AND CONFUCIAN

In their descriptions of affective life over time, my respondents often made clear distinctions between historical periods in Ho Chi Minh City: colonial, socialist, and đổi mới or before and after the "liberation" (giải phóng) of Saigon on April 30, 1975. However, these periods' legacies cannot be so neatly parsed. Rational self-calculation and self-sufficiency can certainly be found in the self in postreform Vietnam, but they are often produced through engagements with socialist and Confucian models of selfhood. Thus, a purely neoliberal, socialist, or Confucian self exists only as idealized forms in Vietnam. People draw from them, sometimes concurrently, to define and redefine themselves (Leshkowich 2022). Together, these multiple strands make up the đổi mới self, a collection of neoliberal, socialist, and Confucian ways of living in Ho Chi Minh City. The đổi mới self is the process of becoming oriented by or toward the marketized values, ethics of personal responsibility, and practices of self-cultivation that have become the hallmarks of neoliberal projects in Vietnam and elsewhere (Rose 1999; Ong and Zhang 2008). The results of this process are contingent on an individual's age, gender, socioeconomic status, and regional background, but although đổi mới selfhood hinges on any number of variables, emotion and sentiment provide a constant terrain for such divergences.

Ironically, the neoliberal construction of the rational self depends on a complementary understanding of the self as emotional and irrational. Despite its having no historical associations with the dichotomy between emotion and cognition, many of my respondents invoked the yin-yang (âm-dương) cosmological theory to explain the supposedly dualistic nature of people's emotional and rational character. Mastery over the self requires recognition of one's susceptibility to emotions in order to identify their threat to rationality, and the more emotion is viewed as a source of self knowledge, the greater the need for self-control becomes. As Minh, a forty-two-year-old former counselor now working as an elementary school teacher, told me, "When a person [is] 'understanding' [the self] then it's easier to 'control'[8] it."[9] Unlike the strategy of remaining silent as a means of self-control discussed in chapter 2, his argument focuses less on an outward expression of the self than on disciplining the inner self through seemingly benign practices of self-exploration. Minh's previous clients' disparate problems to be addressed through self-understanding include marital strife, work difficulties, and conflicts with parents, but what unites them is a resolution through careful consideration of people's own motivations and emotional reactions. In these situations, individuals strategize ways to interact with others and to handle themselves. Disentangling affective states from social life, the imperative to understand the self in order to control it invites reflection on a monadic, autonomous, and sovereign self.

When he was eighteen, Anh left the central coast to major in finance in Ho Chi Minh City and take advantage of its business opportunities but found himself distracted by the city's myriad diversions. Since graduating two years late, he has been unable or unwilling to find employment with enough growth potential to satisfy his parents. Now twenty-five, Anh thinks he is more emotional than most of his peers but draws upon technological metaphors to represent his psyche. His playfully computerized self contains an "A: drive" for himself, a "C: drive" for control, and an "E: drive" for his emotions. Admittedly, his C: drive cannot compensate for his outsized E: drive. For example, he failed some accounting exams because he was too bored to study. The practical advice his friends offered did not mitigate his boredom or heartbreak because, according to Anh, his emotions expressed a fundamental truth about himself and, thus, could (and should) not be restrained. The privileging of *cảm xúc* validates his rejection of others' expectations of how he should prepare for his future, allowing Anh to determine his own.

At first glance, Anh's sense of self corresponds with Western constructions. His formulation of the A:, C:, and E: drives broadly parallels the psychoanalytic tripartite theory of mind that consists of the ego, superego, and id, which he learned from Wikipedia. However, his C: drive contains not only the practices of self-care and governance often associated with neoliberalism, but also practices of sentiment (e.g., calling his parents every week). In relating the superego/C: drive and his parents together, he draws on a practice of sentiment, specifically "checking in" (*hỏi thăm*), to construct his sense of rationality. In doing so, he splits the emotional component from the filial obligations toward his parents as dictated by *tình cảm*. When Anh reluctantly returned to his hometown to take a position in his father's office, he coped with the transition by framing his new life as a test of his mettle that would make him a better person. In effect, he drew upon the imagined powers of the self so often associated with neoliberalism (Ong and Zhang 2008) to fulfill filial obligations. New ways of imagining selfhood create new relationships both to one's self and to others.

In imagining a specific repository for his emotions, Anh objectifies and locates them within the core of his being. At times, he seemed more preoccupied with his emotions than with the objects of those emotions. As a metaphysical substance, emotion constitutes an essence of his self. Assumptions of emotions as discrete entities residing within the self allow him to observe and attempt to control them as if they were detached from him. Ironically, emotions here have a seeming distancing effect on the self; they objectify the self to render it decipherable to him. This reflects the "emotional style" of late capitalism that entails a division between "an intense subjective life and an increasing objectification of the means to express and exchange emotions" (Illouz 2007, 38). By contrast, sentiment cannot be separated from its relational context and underscores its ability to orient individuals to subsequent action by indexing one's relationship to the object of emotion (Shohet 2013).

Although Anh and Hoa are roughly the same age, they have remarkably different affective styles. While their unique personal dispositions account for some of this difference, the class and gender dynamics that impact their access to technologies and regimes of the self are also at play. Anh's parents, who first met as contract laborers in East Germany, have an advantageous political history, allowing his father to find secure employment for himself and his children in a state-owned company. Anh's solidly middle-class position enables him to engage in emotive discourses and puts him at odds with his family, something that Hoa avoided doing at extreme cost to herself. Furthermore, without the gendered expectations of familial care, Anh was given more latitude to pursue a future of his own design. Even when he acquiesced to his parents' demands to return home and care for his ailing father, he framed his circumstances in emotive, not sentimental, terms. Perhaps Hoa would have benefited from following some of Anh's affective lead. Rather than casting her anxieties over moving to the United States as childish and ungrateful, the contemporary discourse of emotion in Vietnam would validate her feelings. However, the extent to which this would have changed her outcome, especially for the better, is unclear. After all, Hoa ultimately lived up to her ambitions while Anh fell short of his.

A self-consciously emotive lens orients people toward a new social and material environment by pluralizing the emotions as well as their objects. In recasting social experience within a rubric of emotion, individuals not only pay more attention to the emotions but modify the concept of emotion itself, such that the criteria for what is considered an "emotion" changes. Categorizing and coding discrete feeling states as emotion means that each of those states inhabits an equal amount of conceptual terrain as each other. That is, anxiety, happiness, and anger are equal to each other in the extent of their "emotion-ness." Conversely, sentiment is a more hierarchically organized social field in which certain cases of sentiment are more important than others and more exemplary of sentiment. The parent-child relationship is the gold standard of a sentimental relationship, while friendships between peers, though valued, are not imbued with the same level of import.

When understood as a natural and value-neutral phenomenon, people link *cảm xúc* with individual freedom and use it to legitimize one's individuality and new social relationships. Attaching to other people as well as objects, practices, and ideas, the possible objects of *cảm xúc* are more inclusive than the more person-oriented notions of *tình cảm*. This horizontal effect produces a sense of the individual self as those feelings' source. The emotivist self is not defined by one's incorporation into social groups; no more authentic version of this self exists beneath such relations. Cutting through the explicitly interpersonal fields of sentiment, *cảm xúc* has become a principal means through which people can understand themselves as fundamentally in conflict with filial obligations and expectations. For example, Anh often clashed over the direction of his career with his father. His primary excuse for increasingly disregarding his father's advice, vocational or otherwise, was that he himself needed to find a calling that he was genuinely passionate about. Taking on this challenge helps Anh understand himself as being able to exercise power over his own self and negotiate his own position in the world. A professional and personal path would follow the discovery of his *sui generis* self.

Looking inward for spiritual growth and subsistence, a self organized by *cảm xúc* takes the heart as both the source and arbiter of moral action. Emotions are conceived as a privileged source of self-understanding. Whereas discourses of *tình cảm* emphasize the obligations people have toward each other, people saw themselves as having "rights" to feel a particular way, irrespective of who or what the object of that emotion is.[10] The balance between these rights and obligations can often seem to tip either way, depending on the purpose it was invoked for. For example, Trâm, a thirty-seven-year-old woman, is old enough to remember the lean years of the immediate postwar subsidy period yet young enough to come of age under *đổi mới*. Despite the gravity of her childhood circumstances, according to her, the biggest crisis of her life was the recent discovery of her husband's extramarital affair. According to her, this shock (*sốc*) was the only justification needed to start an affair of her own if she so desired, but she maintained that she would not follow through with this course of action, out of commitment to her own spousal obligations (*tình nghĩa*). These sentimental duties are the continued responsibilities that spouses are expected to carry out even in loveless marriages. However, when she conducted a brief affair of her own, Trâm blamed her emotions and the capriciousness of the heart. That she experienced tremendous guilt about the matter, despite the assuredness of her prior justification, indicates her own struggle between regimes of emotion, sentiment, and selfhood. We will return to Trâm's dilemmas in chapter 6.

Many Ho Chi Minh City residents frame the self as absorbed in the demands of everyday life, reflecting the individuated subjectivities associated with neoliberalism. Submerging emotional life in the quotidian highlights the personal self at the expense of the national self and its emphasis on heroic socialism.[11] No longer bound to the actions of revolutionary zeal, selfhood is firmly rooted and finds intrinsic meaning in the banalities of family and work life. Moreover, an emphasis on how an individual feels about something shifts from both Confucian and socialist forms of social organization that valorize communality and hierarchy. The breakdown of such institutions is frequently associated with opening new spaces for alternative sources of meaningful content in people's lives.

For example, Thiện, a twenty-three-year-old bank employee, viewed the everyday as the setting in which self-discovery is achieved, even in tragedy. When I ran into him one evening, he was still mulling over a conversation—with Hiếu, his roommate's thirty-eight-year-old brother, and two of Hiếu's friends, a heterosexual couple in their forties—at a café earlier that afternoon. Widowed some months prior, Hiếu had spoken of wanting to remarry in the near future, and his friends advised him on the difficult but important task of finding a suitable woman near his age. Thiện was struck by Hiếu's desire to move on with his life so soon after his wife's death but was even more puzzled by the "strange community" that Hiếu and his friends constituted. How could people of that age and life experience cope with a wife's death simply by replacing her? Why did they not realize that Hiếu needed more time by himself to process his grief? According to Thiện, remarrying so quickly could only be a temporary solution, akin to plugging a few holes in a balloon that would inevitably deflate. Perhaps to find some closure on the matter, he declared them simply to be "not very Vietnamese."

Contrary to Thiện's assessment, however, Hiếu's actions can be construed as falling in line with various Vietnamese traditions. For example, finding another wife would allow him to reestablish a social order that restores his role as a husband who is the provider and public face of his family; the death of a spouse is not just an emotional loss but a loss of social status, and the corrective for this social problem relies on external measures addressing matters of the heart.[12] Moreover, the notion of marriage as a primarily emotional institution in Vietnam is linked to *đổi mới* (Phinney 2008a). Problems are to be resolved, not dwelled upon, in Ho Chi Minh City's actions-speak-louder-than-words spirit. Thus, advice from many family and friends often focuses on the correct course of action based on whatever relationship of sentiment is involved, such that the affective and role correctives are fused.

On the other hand, Thiện's model of proper grieving requires the scrutiny of one's own emotions in order to determine the needs, desires, and contours of the self. From this perspective, Hiếu was only going through the motions of coping with his wife's death—more "mechanical," in Thiện's words, than fully human. Thus, it is Thiện's assumptions about the emotive self that seem "not very Vietnamese." He wondered why the people he was having coffee with had not yet developed the "tools" to understand themselves. Answering the question of how he came to possess them, Thiện joked that he was good at English. His flippant answer points to the relative novelty of *cảm xúc* as a technology of the self in Vietnam. Its power is evident in how Hiếu and his friends were made unrecognizable to Thiện as fellow Vietnamese. Perhaps for Thiện, one of emotion's greatest ironies is that its promise to access a more authentic self may also have estranged him from others, and perhaps even from himself.

CONCLUSION

The current popular interest in emotion in Vietnam contradicts popular assumptions that modernity entails an increased rationalization of the self and desiccation of affective life. Indeed, in the case of East and Southeast Asian neoliberalisms, the emergent self is profoundly emotive. Instead of reductively conceptualizing emotion as either oppositional or epiphenomenal to capitalism, scholarship on neoliberalism in the region has focused on how various emotionally laden practices facilitate the rationalization of the self typically associated with neoliberalism (Skidmore 2003; Jones 2004; Lindquist 2008; Rudnyckyj 2011; Hien 2012). These lines of inquiry suggest that the performance and experience of certain emotions are not only central to the subjective experience of the transition to a market-oriented economy, but also serve as the conduits through which political economies transform selfhood.

In constructing themselves as individuals and as members of the Vietnamese nation through the lens of the emotions, Ho Chi Minh City residents simultaneously make sense of ongoing societal changes and alter the meaning of their individual and collective past. The emergence of emotion as a category to structure the self provides people a different way of imagining both everyday life and one's larger life of significance. Thus, how people conceptualize emotion in relation to their own lives powerfully mediates the production of contemporary selfhood. The elaboration of emotion in Vietnam reconstructs the self in a psychologistic register that is seen as a more accurate mode of self-understanding than ones defined in terms of sentiment. Doing so does not give individuals access to their true, inner selves. Instead, it maps interiority to make it increasingly legible to themselves and others. This process naturalizes regimes of neoliberal, post-socialist statehood and selfhood and creates individuals oriented toward the dynamics of both social and personal transformations. *Cảm xúc* has become an abstracted category that relates a select range of physiological, psychological, and social phenomena to each other and unites them with the common denominator of an inner self. Emotion dialectically constructs the person as an object recognizable to the individual and to others, as well as a self in the process of defining itself through those emotions (Parish 2008).

Part 2 of this book examines the effects of these new regimes of emotion and selfhood on how people understand anxiety in a variety of clinical settings. Whether anxiety is conceptualized in relation to *cảm xúc* or to *tình cảm* influences the way anxiety disorders are diagnosed and treated. However, the rise of an emotive discourse in everyday life in Ho Chi Minh City has implications for anxiety beyond its conceptual and discursive framing. Martha Nussbaum (2001) argues that emotions are judgments of value that attribute importance to things and persons outside of one's own control, effectively acknowledging a lack of self-sufficiency. Certainly, more attention directed toward one's own emotions accords with a neoliberal ethos of self-care. However, along with the recognition of the lack of control over the object of the emotion, emotion perpetually underscores the impossibility of self-sufficiency. As many in Ho Chi Minh City are beginning to realize, this impossibility becomes a defining feature of the self. It also echoes the psychic conditions of the self faced with its own indeterminacy that lead to anxiety. When Ho Chi Minh City residents explore and engage with a fuller range of emotions, are they leaving the door open wider to some affective states than to others?

PART TWO

Clinical Manifestations of Anxiety

4

The Medicalization of Worry

People in Ho Chi Minh City occasionally joke that they live at 766 Võ Văn Kiệt Street in District 5, the address of the Ho Chi Minh City Psychiatric Hospital (*Bệnh viện Tâm thần Thành phố Hồ Chí Minh*). During my early fieldwork, all roads leading there were covered in a thick layer of dust from the repaving of the surrounding neighborhoods. An environmental safety project funded by the Japanese government had partially dredged the Tàu Hủ Channel that runs in front of the hospital grounds, so winds often brought in the scent of the polluted Saigon River. The unruliness of the hospital's exterior, however, is no match for its interior. Hailing from across southern Vietnam, patients and their family members line up hours before the doors open to secure an appointment and then scramble to find space in waiting rooms, hallways, and staircases while they wait as doctors, nurses, administrators, and security guards expertly weave their way past them.[1] Although it still manages to seem like an out-of-the-way place, as the joke about its address attests, the Ho Chi Minh City Psychiatric Hospital looms large in the public imagination. Indeed, the specter of madness itself is also not far from people's minds. Comments and jokes about others or oneself being crazy (*điên*) are routine in everyday conversation, yet admission of one's own mental health struggles is exceedingly rare.

Perhaps it should not have come as a surprise when Vietnam's National Psychiatric Association made headlines in 2017 by announcing that Vietnam faced a mental health crisis hiding in plain sight. According to their estimates, 16 percent of the population could potentially be diagnosed with some form of mental disorder,[2] and roughly forty thousand individuals die by suicide every year (Dương Liễu 2017; Liên Châu 2017).[3] With steadily rising numbers of patients treated at the main psychiatric hospital, Ho Chi Minh City has the highest rates of mental illness in Vietnam. For example, the prevalence of all anxiety disorders in the city is 6.1 percent, compared with 2.27 percent for the rest of the country. Many psychiatrists told me that large swaths of the population are undiagnosed and unwell, requiring treatment to reach their full potential. Instead, they either squandered their opportunities or wasted their money on doctors who were treating essentially psychosomatic symptoms. Reflecting the increased economization of mental health, psychiatrists warned that not treating undiagnosed conditions would be more costly than addressing their needs and positioned themselves as critical to the progress of national development. Increased attention to mental health concerns, however, is not limited to health and development experts. One of the biggest changes I have noticed over the course of my research is the growing awareness and even open discussion of mental health, especially among the younger members of Ho Chi Minh City's middle class.

Most people attribute the surge of mental illness in Vietnam to the destabilizing force of rapid economic growth. This linkage of sweeping social transformations and mental health issues is perhaps the most extreme version of the age of anxiety. The master narratives of modernity's emotional fallout typically blame disruptions in traditional social patterns and relationships that once had a protective effect, changes in people's lifestyles, and greater individual and interpersonal uncertainty as society becomes more dynamic for a number of new social problems, not just increased rates of mental illness (Duong et al. 2011). What these accounts by experts and laypersons have in common is the tangential position of mental illness, especially anxiety disorders, in Vietnam's developmental trajectory. However, development is not just a standardized set of economic benchmarks (Escobar 1991), but also entails their social and emotional impacts. As I have argued in the preceding chapters, anxiety plays a critical role in Vietnam's transition to a market economy. The relationship between mental health and developmental imaginaries shapes the lived context of emergent diagnoses and how they rearticulate long-standing notions of health and the good life.

In Ho Chi Minh City's psychiatric hospitals and clinics, imaginaries surrounding chronic anxiety that articulate various ideals of emotion and selfhood take multiple forms. The most dominant of these is the Western biomedical approach that constructs a broad range of emotional distress as a health problem to be treated with medical intervention. While the use of biomedical diagnoses and treatments outside of the West introduces new perspectives through which to address psychiatric disorder as well as understand the self, it also has the potential to create conflicts between competing traditions of mental health care. Imposing Western standards of normative behavior around the world reduces the personal and cultural meanings of suffering to signs of an underlying disease. This makes people more legible to medical institutions that focus on treating individual symptoms at the expense of recognizing community and state-level factors. The spread of biomedical psychiatry is neither uniform nor inevitable. Indeed, the growing acceptance of diagnoses such as generalized anxiety disorder (GAD), major depressive disorder (MDD), and post-traumatic stress disorder (PTSD) in Vietnam does not necessarily mean that biomedical categories are in the process of replacing preexisting ones. Rather, tensions between competing medical traditions are dynamic, and this chapter presents a portrait of anxiety disorders in Ho Chi Minh City in 2008.

While doctors at the Ho Chi Minh City Psychiatric Hospital usually attribute the various symptoms associated with chronic worry to GAD, their patients identify with a different diagnosis altogether: neurasthenia (*suy nhược thần kinh*, lit. nervous/neurological degeneration).[4] The diagnosis, along with the related notion of *surmenage* (French for "overwork"), has also been recorded among overseas Vietnamese populations and community health workers in Hà Tây Province in northern Vietnam (Phan and Silove 1997; Cheung and Lin 1997; Hinton et al. 2003, 2007; Niemi et al. 2009). My interlocutors regard neurasthenia as a physiological condition caused by an impaired nervous system. Colloquially, the diagnosis also connotes a wide range of psychopathologies, from a delicate psychological constitution to psychosis (Phan and Silove 1999), but here I focus on its anxiety-related components for comparative purposes. Patients' and doctors' medicalizations of anxiety articulate different models of emotion, sentiment, and selfhood in Vietnam. In addition to being a way of enacting obligations of sentiment and moral selfhood, worry is also becoming an emotional obstacle to self-realization.

ANXIOUS IDIOMS OF DISTRESS

Worry-related idioms of distress influence the personal and social meanings of chronic anxiety and treatment seeking (Guarnaccia et al. 2003; Nations et al. 1988), and a proper understanding of them may improve doctor-patient communication and treatment adherence (Hinton and Lewis-Fernandez 2010; Nichter 2010). Complaints of "thinking a lot," for example, frequently index chronic worry (Hinton et al. 2015; Yarris 2011). Anxiety and anxiety disorders may also manifest somatically, such as *chinta rog* (worry illness) in Bangledesh (Rashid 2007), *el calor* among Salvadoran refugees (Jenkins and Valiente 1994), *nervios* in several Latin American populations (Jenkins and Cofresi 1988; Low 1985), and tinnitus and olfactory panic among Cambodian refugees (Hinton et al. 2004, 2006).

Reflecting a medical cosmology that distinguishes between but does not dichotomize mind and body, Vietnamese descriptions of emotional distress frequently invoke somatic states. Worry is associated with weak spleens, loss of appetite, shallow breathing, and stiff necks[5] (Phan and Silove 1999). Frequent orthostatic panic attacks, often induced by standing upright, among traumatized Vietnamese refugees stem from associations between dizziness and memories of physical violence, malaria, or seasickness during attempts to escape Vietnam by boat. Symptomatic of a weak heart, dizziness metaphorically evokes distress and disorder (Hinton et al. 2007). The common syndrome of being "hit by the wind" (*bị trúng gió*) refers to a variety of ailments caused by harmful winds entering the pores of bodies weakened by overworry, insomnia, and thinking a lot (Hinton et al.

2003). Furthermore, nerves serve as both an idiom of distress and a folk illness in rural and peri-urban northern Vietnam (Gammeltoft 1999; Niemi et al. 2013).

NEURASTHENIA

One of the most well-known objects of inquiry in the cross-cultural study of mental illness, neurasthenia has long been analyzed as a somatic idiom of distress for socially unsanctioned emotional problems (Kleinman 1982, 1986; Kleinman and Kleinman 1991; Skultans 1995). Taken together, historical and cross-cultural scholarship on the diagnosis highlights the processes of social interaction that organize perception, emotion, and coping responses around what is most at stake for sufferers, their friends and family, and their healers. As originally defined by the neurologist George Beard in *American Nervousness* (1881), neurasthenia is a chronic disease of the nervous system that manifests as a host of psychic and bodily complaints, including exhaustion, memory loss, sleep disturbance, and various aches and pains, and results from the degeneration of nerve tissue due to overuse. Proclaimed a uniquely "American disease," its popularity among the white upper class was blamed on the pressures of rapid industrialization and urbanization, which took a heavy toll on the swelling numbers of "brain workers" required to maintain the country's new economy. Thus, it encapsulated prevailing concerns about living too fast and the excessive demands for financial and psychic resources in early twentieth-century America (Lutz 1991; Campbell 2007). As neurasthenia became linked to modernity, the development of a neurasthenic American subject became a simultaneous construction of a modern one (Luthra and Wessely 2004).

Despite the purported Americanness of neurasthenia, the diagnosis spread to Europe and its colonies. Colonial officers in the early twentieth century became wary of the vulnerabilities of their positions, succumbing in near-epidemic proportions to "tropical neurasthenia," a lethargic state brought on by an inability to adjust to a climate unfamiliar and unsuitable to Europeans. Furthermore, that only whites received this diagnosis reinforced the idea that the malady was reserved exclusively to those deemed sensitive and cultured enough to suffer from it (Anderson 1997). Whereas neurasthenia in the West was associated with the strains of modern life, tropical neurasthenia was blamed on Westerners' separation from modern civilization and indicated the dangers of administering indigenous populations, thereby emphasizing white civility.

After French officers in colonial Indochina framed tropical neurasthenia as a *malaise de civilisation*, between World Wars I and II, the Vietnamese urban elite began to diagnose themselves as neurasthenic, for two principal reasons. Identifying with neurasthenia suggests an "appropriation from below" in which some Vietnamese individuals characterized themselves as suffering from an excess of civilization (Monnais 2012). The medicalization of anxiety in Vietnam during the 1920s and '30s was both produced by the desire for evidence of civilized modernity, viewed by many Vietnamese as necessary to national independence, and indicative of a growing medicalization of Vietnamese society (Edington 2021). However, since then, the status of neurasthenia in Vietnam as proof of one's own enlightened—if overburdened—state of mind has changed dramatically.

MEDICALIZING WORRY: NEURASTHENIA

Readers familiar with the foundational work of Arthur Kleinman and his associates on neurasthenia in China will recognize broad similarities between the Chinese and Vietnamese cases. A Chinese protectorate from the second century BCE until 938 AD, Vietnam retains Sinitic-derived features in several domains. Most relevant here is the somatopsychic orientation of health in which instances of mental illness are interpreted primarily through bodily symptoms. Chinese medicine (*thuốc bắc*, lit. northern medicine) and Vietnamese medicine (*thuốc nam*, lit. southern medicine; or *thuốc ta*, lit. our medicine) share underlying theories of health, illness, and medicine and are commonly practiced alongside biomedicine throughout Vietnam (Craig 2002; Monnais, Thompson, and Wahlberg 2012). However, while Kleinman's study of China during the 1970s and '80s examined the conceptions of neurasthenia shared by doctors and patients alike,[6] in 2008 only patients at the Ho Chi Minh City Psychiatric Hospital labeled their illness neurasthenia.[7] Most of the patients in the city's public psychiatric hospitals and clinics have lower- or middle-class backgrounds, as wealthy Ho Chi Minh City residents can afford to be treated at private clinics or international hospitals.

Core symptoms of neurasthenia include insomnia (*mất ngủ*), thinking a lot (*suy nghĩ nhiều*), exhaustion (*mệt mỏi*), and headaches (*nhức đầu*). Patients' prioritization of somatic symptoms shaped the quality and interpretation of the experience of neurasthenia into a primarily physiological one, as opposed to the intrapsychic experience of GAD and MDD in the West. Only one of the patients began her foray into professional treatment for her symptoms at a psychiatric clinic. Rather, most patients suffered for years before being referred to the psychiatric hospital by primary-care physicians. Echoing similar findings among overseas Vietnamese populations (Gold 1992; Hinton et al. 2007), psychologically oriented complaints were rarely volunteered and were presented with less frequency and urgency.[8] Indeed, doctors resorted to eliciting information from them with direct yes/no questions about chronic worry, depression, suicidal ideation, and hallucinations. After his appointment, Bình, a fifty-two-year-old man, admitted to me that he did not understand his official diagnosis of depression or what it had to do with his symptoms. Suffering from insomnia for years before seeking treatment, he was unable to fall asleep because he could not stop himself from thinking at night. However, Bình quickly glossed over questions about any sources of sadness or anxiety—both of his sons had substance abuse issues—as if they were irrelevant to his health concerns. A causal link was attributed to his worries, but they were considered a categorically separate domain from the reason for seeking treatment.

Despite the somatopsychic orientation of Vietnamese health beliefs, many patients recognize the psychic basis of their complaints. Regardless, treatment seeking is directed toward physical complaints. The psychological causes of neurasthenia seem detached from many other patients' explanatory models because they were not pathologized. When depressed moods and anxiety were recognized as symptoms, many patients did not tell anybody about them because they were "normal" (bình thường) and "natural" (tự nhiên). Patients who admitted emotional distress rarely identified a specific cause, instead only mentioning a generally stressful situation. The separation of the psychologically oriented etiology from the physiologically oriented frameworks of symptoms and treatments reflects many of the patients' emphasis on their discrete symptoms over an underlying disorder. For example, often used interchangeably with worrying, thinking a lot is blamed by many patients as one of the main reasons for their loss of sleep. Indeed, doctors often ask patients if they had been thinking a lot when probing for anxiety-related symptoms. Yet patients do not seek treatment for cognitive hyperarousal but rather for insomnia. Many doctors even describe benzodiazepines such as Valium and Xanax as sedatives (thuốc ngủ) instead of anxiolytics (thuốc chống lo âu) to their patients to convince them to comply with their prescriptions (Tran et al. 2020).

While biomedical models of mental illness dichotomize mind and body, the Vietnamese medical cosmology posits a more intertwined connection between them (Phan and Silove 1999; Nguyễn 2004). For example, the nervous system connects the workings of the body with the physical environment and conveys feelings such as stress or sadness. Understandings of how strés operates have been mapped onto existing beliefs about worry's impact on the nervous system. However, strés is mostly used in reference to the problems of modern life and does not carry the moral valence of worry. The nerves (dây thần kinh) themselves are a network of fibers that spread outward from the brain and are required to control one's own body and behavior (Craig 2002). Nervousness or tension (căng thẳng) implies nerves stretched to a breaking point (Hinton et al. 2003). Nerves may be compromised by environmental factors (e.g., sudden temperature or wind fluctuations) and by dwelling on distressing matters. Furthermore, descriptions of psychiatric illnesses in Vietnamese medical texts often invoke physical ones (Phan, Steel, and Silove 2004). Phượng, a fifty-seven-year-old inpatient at the Central Psychiatric Hospital II in nearby Biên Hòa, regarded her depression merely as a symptom of neurasthenia, not as her primary diagnosis. She reported that before she became ill she could produce tears when she cried, which would alleviate the felt experience of sadness. However, she had since lost the ability to cry and could only fixate on troubling matters without recourse to the solace provided by crying. Phượng's daughter, who was visiting her, added that Phượng seldom laughed, another marked change. Hence, her chronic anhedonia was interpreted as a "broken" ability to laugh or cry.

Notions of health in Vietnam are explicitly related to strength, emphasizing an internal and stable source of energy and the ability to cope with the everyday stresses of work and a changing environment (Craig 2002). Descriptions of being drained of strength (*hết sức*) imply a finite amount of energy that may or may not be replaced (Hinton et al. 2003). By noting that they were "tired inside the body" (*mệt trong người*), several patients specified that they were exhausted from an internal source instead of from physical activity. Strong nerves, in particular, are associated with vitality, determination, and intelligence—qualities necessary to the fulfillment of family and work obligations (Craig 2002). Conversely, weak nerves put people at risk for a range of maladies, from mild headaches to insanity. Sometimes regarded as a milder version of neurasthenia, the folk illness of nerves (*bệnh thần kinh*) compromises people's capacity to meet their obligations (Gammeltoft 1999). According to the ideal of strong nerves, "healthy individual bodies know how to behave and position themselves socially" (Gammeltoft 1999, 144).

Given the barrage of reasons for their complaints, patients worried about being unable to replenish their energy, strength, and health. For example, Hạnh, a forty-four-year-old marketplace vendor, had a bad fall two years prior to seeking treatment at the psychiatric hospital. The resulting spinal injury forced her, on doctor's orders, to lie down for most of the day for nearly two months. During this time, fears of permanent paralysis led to heart palpitations that continued after her back recovered. She found sleep unrestful, even after sleeping ten hours. These complaints were deemed nonthreatening by a number of cardiologists in Ho Chi Minh City, one of whom told her that her symptoms were merely "neurasthenia of the heart" (*suy nhược thần kinh tim*) and referred her to the psychiatric hospital. That the heart (*tim*, Vietnamese; *tâm*, Sino-Vietnamese) is the traditional locus of the psyche (*tâm lý*, lit. heart and reason) compounded Hạnh's fears of becoming mentally compromised. Physical strength is correlated with an emotional strength that is characterized by resilience is the face of difficulties. Hạnh's hopes focused on regaining the ability to do her work "normally" again, a matter not just of economic productivity and survival but of proper morality as well.

Because moral personhood in Vietnam is enacted through the performance of gendered social roles, many patients like Hạnh describe their exhaustion and weakness in terms of being unable to perform formerly simple activities that are crucial to successful home and work lives. When asked what measures they took to relax, women reported doing household chores to divert themselves from worrisome thoughts.[9] (Conversely, men often resorted to watching TV, reading newspapers, or drinking alcohol as a distraction.) Performing domestic affairs increases women's productivity and contributions to the family but perhaps elides the personal significance and implications of their feelings. Complaints and hopes for recovery are couched in an idiom of social obligations, communicating not only the severity of their symptoms but also their moral standing. Women's symptoms, in particular, are thus inextricable from the gendered emotional labor necessary for families to function properly.

Hạnh's continued concerns over threats of paralysis, restless sleep, and heart palpitations compounded her other worries, including a husband prone to gambling and two feckless adult sons. Despite receiving little comfort or support from them, she continued working long hours in the marketplace to fulfill the sentimental obligations of a wife and mother. Worries about her own health were couched in concerns and disappointments with regard to her family life. Hạnh's husband told her she was worrying needlessly, and I suspected she would agree with this. However, the inability to control her worry and thought processes is what was socially expected of her. Frequent worriers are seen as people who accept the responsibility to be concerned for others and to work to ensure their well-being. For Hạnh, worry is less a symptom or negative coping style, as it is framed within biomedical psychiatry, than a burden that defines her place in the family.

Although neurasthenia diminishes patients' abilities to perform their responsibilities toward their loved ones, the diagnosis still lends them social and moral legitimacy because it is proof of how much they endure for others. Moreover, the emphasis on physical symptoms allows patients to avoid the stigma attached to mental illnesses by legitimizing bodily expressions of emotional distress. Even if aware of anxious or depressive moods, patients may rationalize or hide their emotional problems, given that a person's virtue during periods of suffering is assessed on heroic stoicism. As an ethical practice, endurance without complaint is a form of sacrificing for others that maintains a sociomoral order. This is a conscious decision that patients make, but it also happens through the imagined encouragement or plight of loved ones motivating them to persevere (Gammeltoft 2021). Patients in their twenties and thirties frequently cite caring for their young children as both a cause of anxiety and the reason they did not give up. For Hạnh and Bình, whose grown children did not fulfill their moral duty to reciprocate care for their parents as they got older, this motivation itself must have been a source of strain.

Almost all of the interviewees' ideal course of treatment involved pharmaceuticals. Stemming from the diverse array of tonics and herbal remedies used in Vietnamese and Chinese medicine, treatment preferences emphasize medications for a variety of ailments. Biomedicine is understood to alleviate symptoms but does not cure an illness or address its underlying causes. Moreover, it has powerful short-term efficacy but also comes with more adverse drug reactions than Vietnamese or Chinese medicine (Craig 2002). Thus, recourse to psychopharmaceuticals is seen as an acceptable short-term treatment strategy. That many psychoactive drugs are intended for long-term use undermines adherence to them (Tran 2020).

However, patients recognized that neurasthenia is rooted in social and financial difficulties. Different circumstances would resolve their complaints, and most did not seek out psychiatric care expecting anything other than short-term relief for their physical symptoms. Patients accepted that medication would not remove the stressors that caused and exacerbated their symptoms, in part because there was no expectation that those parts of their lives were under the domain of medical knowledge or mental health. Many had long been modifying their symptoms with prescription medications, supplements, and herbal tonics. These drugs are not aimed at directly transforming the self but instead at supporting it. Indeed, they allow patients to avoid the intense scrutiny of one's own feelings and behaviors within psychotherapy while maintaining their social and moral models of selfhood. That is, patients did not seek pharmaceuticals to mitigate their anxiety. Rather, they wanted medications to reduce their headaches, exhaustion, and insomnia enough that they could worry more, not less.

PSYCHOLOGIZING WORRY: GENERALIZED ANXIETY DISORDER

The Ho Chi Minh City Psychiatric Hospital's outpatient clinic is largely staffed with medical residents eager to put their training into practice and prove their worth as doctors. Many lament the lack of funding for psychiatric services compared to that for other medical specialties in Vietnam, due to pervasive attitudes that psychiatry is more quackery than science. Others had patients who trusted the advice of family members or neighbors more than their own doctors.[10] One strategy of establishing doctors' expertise over patients is discrediting patients' explanatory models. Most doctors at the outpatient clinic were surprised to discover how many of their patients endorsed a diagnosis of neurasthenia and generally dismissed it as a simple problem of health illiteracy. Even common terms for neurasthenia among patients, *suy nghĩ thần kinh* (nervous thinking) and *suy yếu thần kinh* (nervous weakness), were indicative of the extent of the nationwide lack of proper education about psychiatry because these were, according to one resident, not "real words." At best, in this view, patients merely misspoke or misremembered the proper term. Upon learning of patients' identification with neurasthenia, Dr. Quang, thirty-six, segued into a discussion of how rural patients attributed psychiatric problems to ghosts and resorted to herbal remedies or amulets before consulting a physician. That he implicitly grouped the diagnosis with spirit possession and other forms of Vietnamese "superstition" is ironic, since neurasthenia is an American invention. Once embodied as evidence of civilized modernity in Vietnam, neurasthenia has become proof of people's backwardness.

Cross-cultural studies on the tension between biomedical practitioners' and patients' understandings of sickness often frame it as the difference between a system of knowledge that is Western, rational, and scientific and one that is local, meaningful, and symbolic. However, although patient's models of neurasthenia are influenced by Vietnamese medical beliefs, this dichotomy is not applicable here, since both GAD and neurasthenia have biomedical origins. Rather, the primary difference between how patients' symptoms are understood lies not just in the medicalization of worry but also in its psychologization, which Yang (2013, 294) defines as "managing socioeconomic issues in psychological terms." Cartesian models of selfhood posit an individual's private thoughts and feelings as the locus of personal identity (Tran 2017). Moreover, that the only three patients (one woman and two men) in the study who endorsed their official diagnoses of MDD or GAD are in their twenties reflects generational changes in ways of defining the self. However, that their explanatory models did not differ markedly from explanatory models of neurasthenia suggests that these diagnoses are not mutually exclusive for patients. The cultivation of emotional awareness and reflexivity reflects the imperative found in many neoliberalizing economies to encourage personal responsibility and self-management (Zhang 2014; Yang 2014). This project of self-realization assumes that its emancipatory potential comes from exercising individual agency and choice.

However, these undertakings are aimed most directly at Ho Chi Minh City's middle and upper classes. GAD operates on a liberal theory of emotion as something that individuals can possess and therefore control. Both doctors and patients medicalize anxiety, but only the former casts it in a self-reflexively psychologistic register. In contrast to the notions of sentiment that frame worry as a social obligation that individuals must endure, doctors' models of emotion cast worry as personal feeling that individuals must learn to manage. Furthermore, within biomedical psychiatric discourse, individuals who are more attuned to themselves are supposedly better able to create "emotionally democratic" relationships and be independent enough to help themselves and others (Furedi 2004). By highlighting emotion as the crux of patients' illness experience, GAD invites patients to consider their feelings, their causes, and their consequences with the self at the center of their own analysis.

Doctors told me that one of their main tasks is to properly educate patients about their illness. However, most of their efforts to do so are directed at younger and middle-class patients who, they believe, are capable of understanding the diagnosis. In order to properly medicalize their suffering, patients would need to frame their symptoms as underlying GAD and to understand their distress in terms of their own emotions so that they could address the conditions in their lives that led to chronic anxiety. Doctors assumed that with the proper knowledge and tools, patients could properly transform themselves into self-aware and self-sufficient individuals. For example, after finishing a diagnostic interview, Dr. Hùng continued making typical small talk before asking a patient in her twenties what she wanted out of life. She told him that she didn't know repeatedly, until he tried a new strategy. Dr. Hùng chided her for not knowing what she wanted. "How could you not know? It's simple!" He told her she needed to take a step back from her situation and figure out what she wanted. To this she responded, "I don't know how." The transition from "I don't know" to "I don't know how" is revealing: the former is a relatively simple declaration—an admission that the patient did not have a piece of information—but the latter is focused inwardly and highlights a deficiency not just of knowledge but of the self. What brings it about is the doctor's invocation of a new technique of the self: to search her feelings for the answer.

However, within contemporary biomedical psychiatry, patients are increasingly not the experts of their own emotions (Furedi 2004). Often prescribing benzodiazepines or serotonergic antidepressants for GAD and MDD, some doctors at the outpatient clinic occasionally advise patients to seek the counseling services upstairs from the outpatient clinic, where they would be encouraged to engage in further self-analysis. Others, however, dismissed psychotherapy as "just talking" (nói chuyện thôi) to their patients. According to both psychiatrists and psychotherapists, patients with an intimate understanding of their interior lives are more able to control the self. Stressors as disparate as household or workplace conflicts are addressed through a meticulous reflection of individual motivations and reactions. Both doctors and counselors assumed that patients' emotional issues are always present, if latent; and doctors assured me that rates of psychosomatization (tâm thể hóa) throughout the country were high and that nonpsychiatric hospitals were needlessly clogged with people who actually needed psychiatric care. (No official statistics, however, are available to substantiate their claims.) For them, the core of patients' illness experience is defined largely by its emotional qualities.

However, doctors do allow patients' socioeconomic circumstances to guide the diagnostic interview, despite GAD's diagnostic criteria. In its earliest forms in the DSM-III, GAD could be applied to anyone suffering from persistent anxiety for a given period because the criteria did not require that the anxiety be disproportionate in intensity to its cause (Horwitz and Wakefield 2012). Its later iterations require that anxieties not be rooted to a situational reason. That is, anxiety is pathological only if it is deemed "for no good reason." While insisting to me that GAD could be the result of any number of causes regardless of their validity, doctors explicitly honed in on potential causes to hasten the process. For example, questions about marital status or the age of patients' children served as proxies for worries related to spousal conflicts or school tuition, respectively. These inquiries recognize and legitimize patients' refusal to disentangle worry from its social context. One of the most common criticisms of biomedical psychiatry is that it medicalizes people's suffering and ignores the experiential richness of their illness. Indeed, the rise of psychopharmaceuticals over other psychotherapeutic measures as a primary form of treatment is often associated with an emphasis on biological processes over a rich network of meanings used in the healing process. However, in the clinical encounters at the outpatient clinic, the doctors advocate complex understandings of the illness experience that draw from patients' personal lives and social contexts; it is the patients who medicalize their illness in a manner that minimizes the significance of their feelings.

CONCLUSION

While biomedical frameworks of anxiety and anxiety disorders assume their universality (Hinton and Good 2009; Horwitz and Wakefield 2012), attending to their sociocultural and political-economic contexts provides a more nuanced conceptualization of normative and pathological forms of anxiety. The notions of worry, weakness, and health that are expressed in the explanatory model of neurasthenia shape the experience and interpretation of anxiety by relating moral selfhood to distress and disorder. Conceptualizing worry through the lens of sentiment or emotion and as neurasthenia or GAD gives patients and doctors, respectively, different models of and possibilities for the self. Doctors assume that redefining selfhood in emotive terms is a more accurate mode of self-understanding than one defined by relations of sentiment. According to them, accepting the diagnosis of GAD better equips patients to control their emotions and themselves, a purportedly empowering step toward improving their lives. In doing so, they are freed from the constraints of their sentimental ties and transformed into modern subjects (Rose 2006). However, as articulated in clinical settings, these powers of the self are contradicted by the ways the self is marked by vulnerability. When the trials of everyday life take their toll and, in turn, are psychologized and pathologized by biomedical discourses, the emotive self is constructed as a source of power that is inherently vulnerable—a vulnerability that increasingly can be addressed only by biomedical expertise (Illouz 2008).

Although doctors dichotomized GAD as modern and neurasthenia as backwards, patients' understandings of neurasthenia and GAD are not mutually exclusive. Many patients are indeed aware of and want to manage their emotions and their selves, but do so for the purposes of maintaining their own moral integrity and sentimental bonds to others. As distinct yet complementary diagnoses, neurasthenia and GAD complicate notions that Ho Chi Minh City's "age of anxiety" is the result of modernist narratives of progress. For many patients, neurasthenia is more meaningful than GAD because the treatment pertains to their model of disease. Emotional problems are not considered a medical domain, let alone something to discuss with a doctor. Because the primary sources of worry are deemed unresolvable, treating neurasthenia is a way to at least reduce the suffering of patients who are willing to endure some of it. Anxiety itself is too closely intertwined with its causes to be treated or even medicalized and pathologized to begin with. Thus, it is not a symptom of mental illness but an appropriate response to difficult circumstances. In the context of neurasthenia, worry cannot be fixed by medication or self-work because it is knitted into structured hierarchies, relations, and obligations. While the proximate cause of neurasthenia is related to depleted nerves, its ultimate cause is attributed by patients to social conditions, reflecting an approach to psychiatry found throughout East Asia that emphasizes intrapersonal factors less than biomedical ones (Borovoy 2005; Kitanaka 2012; Ma 2012).

Instead of seeking agency in an individuated selfhood, patients draw on a moral discourse of sentiment to frame neurasthenia as a testament to their care and concern for others. Lee (2011) argues that contemporary biomedical diagnoses replaced neurasthenia as a diagnostic entity in China because explicit emotional expression has become more socially acceptable; in this era of "emotional liberalization," people find it easier to express their suffering in the psychologically oriented idiom of depression. However, among the lower-class patients I spoke to at the Ho Chi Minh City Psychiatric Hospital, the very conceptualization of emotion, not its expression, prevented them from readily embracing GAD. Their doctors advocated broad mental health outreach, especially in rural areas, to improve biomedical literacy and correct patient perspectives on psychiatric diagnoses. On a case-by-case basis, however, they rarely explained GAD to lower-class patients and instead stressed the importance of drug compliance. After all, most of the patients were more keen to discuss their medications than their emotional problems. However, this shared focus on pharmaceuticals allowed patients to bypass the self-analysis that the doctors theoretically endorsed. What the doctors did not seem to understand is that the widespread acceptance of GAD as a diagnosis requires changing not just how patients understand anxiety disorders, but also how they understand anxiety itself.

Võ Văn Kiệt Street is now a six-lane highway, making the Ho Chi Minh City Psychiatric Hospital a lot easier to access. Much-needed renovations of the building have also been completed, most notably the removal of the inpatient ward's iron bars, a legacy of the hospital's former use as a colonial prison. Changes have not been limited to the hospital's material structure and surroundings. When I returned for follow-up research less than a decade later, not a single patient mentioned neurasthenia (Tran et al. 2020). Instead, they spoke of GAD and MDD. Any death knells for neurasthenia in Vietnam, however, are likely premature, as the famously protean diagnosis has long been readily adapted to address new sources and forms of modernity's ailments (Bhola and Chaturvedi 2020). Regardless, presuming that the turn toward more contemporary biomedical diagnoses goes beyond a simple terminological update, this shift implies that a broad reconfiguration of the self is under way for many Ho Chi Minh City residents.

5

The Psychologization of Worry

"How much of my job is teaching people how to feel?" Kim, a forty-eight-year-old Vietnamese Australian psychotherapist, asked me in correct anticipation of my next interview question. "One hundred percent." She was joking, but the punch line is worth further consideration. Kim finds that her Vietnamese clients tended to be either completely closed to their emotions or entirely beholden to them. Her mission is to guide them toward a middle ground. The psychotherapeutic process is oriented toward the simultaneous cultivation of an awareness of one's own emotions and the means to discipline them. "It's about emotional regulation," Kim said. Teaching people how to feel "is basically what a counselor is."

Vietnam's age of anxiety has been good for business at Ho Chi Minh City's psychotherapy centers. According to Aaron, an American director of one center, anxiety brings 60–70 percent of clients to his office door. Once there, people are taught a variety of techniques to manage their worries. In doing so, they also learn to reconceptualize their worries in an emotive register as a matter of self-understanding (*hiểu mình* or *xem mình*, lit. observing or considering the self). While doctors at the psychiatric hospital expend most of their efforts on ensuring adherence to medication prescriptions and pay little attention to patients' models of selfhood, psychotherapists often target the self directly in their treatments for anxiety. This process reflects the psychologization of distress, in which the psy-disciplines are marshalled to analyze conditions that are simultaneously psychological, social, and material. Psychotherapy is largely premised on Western, especially North American, notions of the person that valorize individualism, self-fulfillment, and emotional expressiveness, where a richly articulated and layered sense of inner self is evidence of self-coherence (Jenkins and Barrett 2004; Kirmayer and Raikhel 2009; Kirmayer 2007). Thus, going to therapy in Vietnam is about much more than the alleviation of emotional pain. Kim and Aaron's clients may not learn to feel for the first time, but they are taught that some ways of feeling are better than others.

Hailing from Vietnam, the West, and the Vietnamese diaspora in the West, Ho Chi Minh City's psy-experts form an expanding professional network of clinical psychologists, counselors, social workers, applied behavioral analysts, speech and language pathologists, and special education teachers, among others. As such, their interactions with each other can be marked by tensions and disagreements, but what unites them is a shared mission to address a long-ignored treatment gap. Their perspectives on their work and the current state of feeling in Vietnam reflect and reproduce Western discourses of the self that people use to manage themselves in the global economy. Yet many of them are aware of, and conflicted about, the Western bias of their treatments. (Ironically, the Westerners stated more concerns about cultural competence than their Vietnamese counterparts.) Thus, mental health experts cannot be reduced to vectors of self-responsibility. Unlike the psychiatrists and their patients in chapter 4, psychotherapists and their clients increasingly share similar ideals of selfhood if not the same ideas on how to achieve them. Indeed, many of the therapists I spoke with were once clients themselves. They were inspired to their vocation because psychology gave them new ways to understand themselves and others. Ngọc Bình, the popular therapist influencer on TikTok, notes that his training made him more empathetic, so when people share their problems with him, he listens carefully rather than resorting to clichéd words of support (Chi Mai 2021). Many of the people in this book, including Anh (chapter 1), Hoa (chapter 2), and Trâm and Hải (chapter 6), were dissatisfied with the well-meaning but ultimately cold comfort they got from friends and family. Had they consulted with a skilled psychotherapist, they likely would have gained new insights about themselves. However, the impulse to treat therapy as a panacea for so many problems in the world stems from a growing emotionalization of society that assesses crisis primarily by its emotional impacts (Lerner and Rivkin-Fish 2021).

Operating as a global emotion pedagogy that frames the emotions as "teachable skill bundles" (Wilce and Fenigsen 2016, 83), cognitive behavioral therapy (CBT) has become by far the most common form of psychotherapy in the world. However, it has been analytically overlooked in the medical social sciences and humanities.[1] Compared to psychoanalysis (Obeyesekere 1990), family constellations therapy (Pritzker and Duncan 2019), or indigenous and hybrid forms of psychotherapy (Yang 2017), CBT can seem relatively bureaucratic and mechanistic, due to a narrow focus on modifying problematic behaviors. It is explicitly not designed to be exploratory. Yet CBT also rests on a theory of an integrated and egocentric self that must be in place for the treatment to be productively implemented. While CBT's customizable focus on specific issues may be more accessible for Vietnamese clients than the more comprehensive approach of psychoanalysis, the very work of self-compartmentalization requires a broader questioning of personal and cultural identity as therapists and clients alike negotiate the cultural forms that assist and resist the acceptance of psychotherapeutic principles. As the emotions increasingly stand in for some core aspect of people's most authentic self among Ho Chi Minh City's middle class (see chapter 3), discovering the self and controlling it become inextricable. Neoliberal discourses of emotion frame the self as simultaneously capable of self-empowerment and vulnerable to emotional excess (Duncan 2017). A therapeutic monitoring of one's feelings is no longer reserved for disordered minds.

Critics charge that the rise of therapeutic governance in the West indicates a dystopian seizure of people's hearts and minds by the state (Rose 2006; Szasz 2001). Such sweeping claims, however, overlook the negotiations that characterize the spread of the psy-disciplines in the Global South. Focusing on the diverse array of techniques, expertise, and values that produce political subjects outside of the West sheds insight on why certain technologies of the self may be accepted, adapted, or rejected. Thus, rather than frame the globalization of psychotherapy as a simple clash between the traditional and the modern, the rising popularity of psychotherapy in Vietnam and elsewhere suggests an ambivalent terrain upon which people experience the transition to a market economy (Zhang 2017; Matza 2018). While Ho Chi Minh City residents work toward what their psychotherapists view as a modern mindset by engaging with neoliberal discourses of the self, this process does not yield uniform results. For many clients, the motivation to seek treatment stems from desires to reduce intra-family conflict and to retrench relational forms of selfhood instead of replacing them. Thus, psychotherapeutic practices are part of an increasingly diverse set of technologies of the self available to people as they adopt multiple regimes of selfhood. While they certainly differ, such configurations of the self do not necessarily compete against each other. Rather, they are cumulative, expanding the repertoire of possible selves for Ho Chi Minh City residents. Therapeutic selfhood can be simultaneously social and reflexive, private and public, and neoliberal and socialist (Zhang 2018, 2020).

PSYCHO-BOOM-TIMES

That psychotherapy centers even exist in Ho Chi Minh City is notable in a country where Western psychological and behavioral sciences have been contested for much of the twentieth century. During the early colonial period, psychological theories from the West found a receptive audience among the cosmopolitan elites in urban Vietnam, but after World War I, leading Vietnamese intellectuals agitating for national independence favored the political philosophies of Locke, Rousseau, Marx, and Engels (Marr 2000). Meanwhile, French psychiatrists—and, eventually, their Vietnamese counterparts in the colonial asylums—pioneered several therapeutic approaches that became widespread, not just in other colonial holdings in Southeast Asia but in the metropole as well (Edington 2019). For example, bridging the divide between the asylum and its surrounds, racialized notions of labor therapy were designed to prepare patients for life after discharge and instill self-discipline by having them perform agricultural labor. The contemporary psycho-boom is also notable because it contrasts so starkly with the socialist critique of academic psychology as an interest of the self-obsessed bourgeoisie. Throughout the socialist world, psychiatry was generally reserved for addressing psychotic episodes, and mental illness was blamed on erroneous political convictions that were to be treated through "thought work" (cf. Zhang 2018; Huang 2014, 2015). However, in twenty-first-century Vietnam, conversations with foreign discourses of society, civilization, and selfhood have taken a decidedly psychological turn.

Early therapeutic interventions under đổi mới more closely resembled life coaching or training than the psychotherapy typical in the West. This stemmed from many therapists' inclination to provide quick and pragmatic solutions and clients' demands for direct answers to their issues. Members of the first generation of counselors in Vietnam are notorious among the younger therapists I spoke with for only dispensing advice, instead of listening to their clients. As part of their work at an international NGO, Julien and Sylvie, two recently graduated psychotherapists, treated patients and provided training and consulting in psychotherapy at several public hospitals throughout Ho Chi Minh City. They found that the most challenging aspect of their work was in getting Vietnamese mental health specialists to reflect on their own emotional reactions to their patients (i.e., countertransference), beyond whether or not they liked the patients. One counselor at the Ho Chi Minh City Psychiatric Hospital was surprised when Julien criticized her for offering too much advice to a patient and, indeed, for talking more than her patients during their sessions. Instead, like the psychiatrists, these psychologists preferred to focus on helping clients with concrete advice.

Tâm, a sixty-five-year-old woman, founded one of Ho Chi Minh City's first counseling centers in 1997 to apply the insights of psychotherapy and educational psychology to people's sentimental lives (đời sống tình cảm). Her center's primary work revolved around resolving conflicts within marriages, families, and friendships and addressing "social problems" related to domestic violence, gender inequality, and sex and sexuality. Additionally, she was regularly invited to student assemblies at universities to discuss and answer questions related to sexual and reproductive health. Counseling services took place in a spacious room with several desks and folding chairs, cordoned off with paneled room dividers. Most of the clients phoned in for services, so privacy was usually not a significant concern, but if multiple clients were in the center at the same time, an employee would simply open a window to allow the ambient traffic noise to drown out the consultation. A reexamination of the self was not a priority for Tâm and her employees. For example, if a client wanted a divorce from her husband, counselors would encourage them to sacrifice for their children. Their preference for concrete advice over abstract and ponderous self-exploration echoes the thought work promoted by the state to impart socialist ideology to citizens. Indeed, the center's guiding philosophy was inspired by state discourses on proper morality and the "happy family" campaign (cf. Kwiatkowski 2016; Shohet 2017).

Today, psychotherapeutic concepts and techniques are no longer confined to clinical and academic settings. Instead, driven by market demands, they have been flexibly deployed across a wide variety of settings that Ho Chi Minh City's middle class deems in need of psychological intervention. Self-help books in English and in translation sit alongside financial advice books on local bookstore shelves. Schools and corporations incorporate psychotherapeutic techniques to manage their students and employees, and it is not uncommon to see people reading popular psychology books by themselves at cafés. (Ten years ago, it was rare even to see anyone by themselves at a café!) Organized by therapists to supplement their income, paid seminars with psychoeducational themes (stress management, emotional intelligence, introverts vs. extroverts, etc.) are increasingly popular among young professionals, especially those working in human resources, on the lookout for expertise and counsel for their personal and career ambitions as well as networking opportunities. The rise of the psychotherapeutic industry in Vietnam parallels trends elsewhere in the region. For example, China's national certification program in counseling psychology has licensed many within the new middle class (Zhang 2018). Few, however, intend to become mental health professionals. Rather, they are attracted to the courses by the potential to self-actualize an ideal of the good life.

Despite growing popular demand for psychotherapeutic services in Vietnam, thus far the state has offered little support. For example, the national labor code does not recognize psychotherapist as an official occupation, a bureaucratic headache for the growing number of psychotherapists. The lack of government support for and oversight of psychotherapy has led to an unregulated market of counseling services. Freelance counselors range from foreigners seeking to accrue experience for their credentials before returning to their home countries, to both Vietnamese and expatriates with limited training who promise unrealistic outcomes through unorthodox methods (e.g., curing autism with yoga), to a naive clientele largely unfamiliar with the conventions of the field. Kim's husband quipped to her that Westerners can "come to Vietnam and become doctors." By the time that clients or their families realize that such treatments may be more harmful than helpful, their conditions have often worsened to the point where emergency procedures are required. Medical evacuation to inpatient treatment facilities in Singapore or Hong Kong is not uncommon in cases that involve suicidal ideation or prescription drug abuse.

Over the past decade, however, what was once a cottage industry has developed a disciplinary identity with its own set of norms and standards, and the field's increased professionalization has routed out many of the more dubious practitioners. Ten years ago, my conversations with the staff at fledgling counseling centers in Ho Chi Minh City were marked by an undercurrent of embarrassment that someone was even paying attention to them and their work. They emphasized how new the concept of psychotherapy was to Vietnam, as if to apologize for the state of their field. Today's generation of therapists, however, speak with much more assurance and conviction about their work and repeatedly stress the optimistic outlook of their profession. Many spoke of a "big market" for psychotherapy that remains untapped. Tuấn, a fifty-six-year-old clinical psychologist who trained in the United States, wanted to duplicate the success of Chinese private mental health treatment facilities that used a "properly American style" of care in Vietnam. As he told potential capital investors for his own center, "For sure we'll kill it. People are waiting."

COGNITIVE BEHAVIORAL THERAPY IN THEORY

Cognitive behavioral therapy refers to a set of psychotherapeutic approaches developed as an alternative to then-dominant psychoanalytic schools of thought that were increasingly under fire for being too nebulous and time-intensive. During the 1950s, early advocates of behavioral therapy in the United States emphasized scientifically validated techniques rooted in the classical and operant conditioning principles of behaviorism. By the 1970s, the rise of cognitivism and cognitive therapy emphasized the impact of mental phenomena such as thoughts, feelings, and internal reflection on human behavior. Integrating these two approaches as cognitive behavioral therapy focuses on an individual's thoughts and beliefs in order to reduce unwanted behaviors. Oriented toward concrete problems and solutions, CBT is based on the assumption that the development of new coping strategies and ways of processing information blunts the impact of maladaptive thinking, what are called "cognitive distortions." Examples of cognitive distortions include magnifying negative information, minimizing positive information, and catastrophic thinking. The goal of CBT is not so much to diagnose any given disorder but rather to examine specific problems in relation to an individual's life. CBT requires both client and therapist to be actively involved in identifying cognitive distortions and some of the patient's most problematic cognitive and behavioral patterns, as well as developing a strategy to resolve them.

CBT's pragmatic and supposedly atheoretical orientation has contributed to its wide-ranging appeal. Its current prevalence is additionally driven by a user-friendly design with clearly defined techniques that require less extensive training than psychoanalysis. Because the process is driven by concrete strategies, CBT is also fairly easy to standardize in training manuals and commoditize in self-help books. This standardization allows CBT to be tested in efficacy experiments, and its association with evidence-based practices and the scientific method gives CBT the presumption of being value neutral and a seemingly universal applicability.

With the waning popularity of psychodynamic approaches, CBT has become easily the most common evidence-based psychosocial therapeutic practice. Perhaps more critical to CBT's success than its theoretical innovation, however, is its methodological and procedural one. While psychodynamically oriented talk therapy typically requires weekly or biweekly sessions for one to two years to surface the unconscious problems that patients continually stumble on, CBT is short term and goal oriented. Individuals come in once every two or three weeks for four to seven months, for an average of twelve to twenty sessions. As part of the co-construction of the psychotherapeutic practice, therapists and patients devise an action plan, with the patients assigned "homework"—frequently a recording of their thoughts, feelings, and actions to be brought in and analyzed with the therapist.

However, with its therapeutic emphasis on cognition, verbal skills, and rational (however *rational* is defined) thinking, CBT is as value-laden as any form of psychotherapy. Indeed, Euro-American ideals of self and personhood are reflected in a therapeutic emphasis on assertiveness over indirectness and subtlety in social interaction, change over patience and acceptance, personal independence over interdependence, and open self-disclosure over protection of family reputation (Hays 2009). For example, the goal of changing aspects of the inner self assumes that people will assume control over problems such as disturbing thoughts or maladaptive and self-defeating behaviors if they recognize their cognitive distortions and change them to be more helpful, positive, and realistic. However, CBT's individualism and internal locus of control may come into conflict with social and familial hierarchies found throughout East and Southeast Asia (Iwamasa, Hsia, and Hinton 2019). Thus, multicultural psychologists warn CBT practitioners against attributing environmentally based problems to some kind of deficiency in the individual (Hays 2009). As an alternative, Hwang et al. (2006) advise psychotherapists working with minority populations to "acknowledge the discrepancies in cultural expectations and reframe the goals of treatment to developing 'adaptation skills' that are necessary for a healthy life" in order to allow clients to "play out their bicultural selves" (298). According to them, CBT should be adapted—or at least framed differently—for the client. However, when CBT is deployed outside of its native context, a different sort of adaptation occurs.

COGNITIVE BEHAVIORAL THERAPY IN PRACTICE

The PsyCafe's actual café generated little of its revenue. Its primary function was to serve as a cover for privacy-seeking individuals who would proceed upstairs for psychotherapy sessions. Each of the consultation rooms had only enough space for two armchairs, facilitating intimacy between therapist and client. The PsyCafe did have a large seminar room reserved for business meetings and training courses. Every few weeks, Bảo, the fifty-three-year-old owner who was trained as a counselor in Thailand, and a group of five to ten students convened to discuss theory, methodology, and case studies; gather feedback and advise on the students' own clients; and occasionally observe a session with one of Bảo's clients. Almost all the PsyCafe students I met during my research were women. This reflects gender roles that assign women more expectations of care and emotional sensitivity but less pressure to be financially successful, which allows them to pursue their own career interests, so long as they do not interfere with domestic responsibilities.[2] The students range from current and recently graduated college students who want to enhance their training to working professionals who want to maintain their professional and personal ties to each other. Classes typically started with a recap and discussion of the core theoretical tenets of counseling psychology, especially CBT, and workshopping of various cases the students had taken on. Students often referred to CBT simply as *điều trị hành vi* (behavioral therapy), and Bảo had to remind them that the cognitive and behavioral components of the therapy must be linked.

One of the students, a thirty-one-year-old school counselor named Vi, told her classmates about the case of an ethnic Chinese man who consulted her because of his son's frequent disobedience. Corporal punishment is regularly used to discipline boys in Vietnam (Rydström 2006a), but because the son had epilepsy, his parents agreed to never hit him, for fear of triggering a seizure. The central issue that Vi wanted to discuss, however, was not the child but the father.[3] When she asked him to clarify why he wanted his son to be more obedient (*ngoan*), he only repeated that he wanted his son to be similar to a neighbor's more docile child. Regarded as the "pillars" of the Vietnamese family, fathers tend to have an authoritative parenting style, and the man told Vi that a father's commands to his son should be carried out without question or justification. When Vi probed her client about his emotions (*cảm xúc*) regarding the situation, he responded, "What's a feeling?" To this, the rest of the students laughed knowingly at one another. According to Vi, the man did not know if he was sad or not and could only repeat his desire for a more obedient child. One of the students floated the idea that he did not understand the word *cảm xúc* because he is Chinese, but Vi noted that he was born and raised in Vietnam and did not speak Vietnamese with a foreign accent. Others wondered if he simply lacked the habit of talking about his emotions or even lacked any emotions. The lack of emotional awareness already presents a difficult challenge for psychotherapists, but where do Vi and her classmates begin for clients who apparently are not even aware of the concept of emotion?

When asked to account for the relative success of CBT in comparison to other forms of psychotherapy in Vietnam, most mental health experts argued that the appeal lies in both its matter-of-factness and its emphasis on external behavior instead of inner feelings. First, clients often came to treatment with clear goals and direct requests to eliminate their symptoms or change their children's behavior in two weeks. Nguyên, a thirty-year-old counselor at a call-in center in Ho Chi Minh City, observed that his clients' expectation that a single session will yield the advice that will resolve their problems follows a medical model. The explanation that CBT is popular because of a focus on specific problems and quick results is certainly not limited to Vietnam.[4] The specific therapeutic strategies of

CBT reflect the punctuated timeline of late capitalism (Craciun 2016), and the fast pace that many Ho Chi Minh City residents regard as emblematic of a modern lifestyle leaves precious little time for oneself or others.[5] Kim promotes short-term strategies because so many of her clients tend to disappear after a few visits. Her rationale for doing so is that some small adjustments (e.g., doing breathing exercises fives times per day) to the clients' lives would be better than nothing. In some ways, she noted, current trends in psychology, such as the growing popularity of online listicles with titles like "5-Things-To-Do-To-Not-Be-Depressed," jibes with a Vietnamese context, especially in regard to a distinct orientation to behavior.

Second, CBT's perceived emphasis on observable behavior accords with a widespread belief among clients that actions speak louder than words. Ho Chi Minh City residents often noted to me that a person's most authentic self would be revealed in their behaviors. That is, one should not trust what people say but watch what they do. In general, I found most of the people I encountered during my fieldwork to be careful watchers of other people's behaviors, since anticipating others' needs and desires indicates one's own degree of care. Indeed, other people are often regarded as better judges of one's character than one's own self. Moreover, when people recount a story, they tend to describe in detail people's actions, rather than their perceived emotional states. This reflects a perspective on selfhood that emphasizes how one is perceived by others over how one perceives one's own self. Indeed, this greater comfort with behavior is common among many mental health workers as well. According to Julien, CBT has a pragmatically American character that especially appeals to Vietnamese mental health professionals. Hằng, a twenty-nine-year-old applied behavioral analyst who specializes in autism treatment, said that modifying behavior was simply more real. According to her, everything else was "just advice." To effect substantive change in people's lives, an action plan must be applied. Many cognitive-behavioral therapists bristle at the common parlance for a psychotherapist, *bác sĩ tâm lý* (head doctor, lit. psychological doctor), because it evokes notions not dissimilar to the English pejorative *shrink*. Unsurprisingly, they generally disregard psychoanalytically rooted practice, and they also differentiate themselves from other, similarly behaviorally focused mental health experts, such as the applied behavioral analysts. Usually trained in a single narrow specialization, applied behavioral analysts are more akin to technicians and lack the artistry of more broadly trained psychotherapists who can resort to other psychotherapies, even psychoanalysis, when appropriate.

Although familiarity with analyzing observable behaviors, as opposed to subjective experiences, may bring people to the door of the psychotherapy center, it is also what makes the job of a CBT practitioner so difficult. Focusing on behavioral adjustments seems like a convenient way to avoid the difficult work of self-reflection and articulation of interior conflicts. Like the psychiatric patients who only want a drug prescription to treat their anxieties, many clients undergo psychotherapy for instructions on improving their lives or fixing behavioral problems that disrupt family harmony. This echoes a Confucian morality with clearly defined familial roles and the heavy hand of the Vietnamese Communist Party's directions on how to be a good socialist (e.g., remember the fatherland, have no more than two children). However, the neoliberal imperative to be free directs individuals to determine their own path to authentic selfhood without any explicit instructions. Clients are attracted to the medical model of psychiatry because it seems black-and-white to them, but psychotherapy is about, in Julien's words, the complexity of the gray area.

The apparent lack of emotional awareness among many Vietnamese is at the root of both the appeal and the mission of CBT in Vietnam. While emotion is not the primary focus of cognitive-behavioral therapy, CBT theory holds that some degree of emotional reflexivity is necessary so that clients can recognize, if not the psychodynamic roots of their problems, then at least how their problems manifest. Kim says that she "completely understand[s] where they're coming from." She tells her clients that she grew up in Vietnam like them but is upfront about her Western training and methods. She also specifies that they can pick and choose what techniques work or do not work for them, "based on their culture." According to Kim, in the West, therapy is a process of learning, growing, and self-discovery, but in Vietnam people are more problem- and solution-oriented. When her clients ask her point-blank questions on how to solve their problems, they want a prescription in terms of both pharmaceutical and psychosocial treatments.

For example, when Kim explained the symptoms of PTSD to a woman in her twenties who suffered from trauma-induced nightmares and panic attacks, the client asked, "Can I just forget this?" Whereas Kim's clients in Australia sought to process their trauma and earn something from it, this patient effectively wanted to learn how to walk away from it without confronting it directly. According to Kim, Westerners are more indulgent in their suffering and want to "dump it out on someone else" in order to work through it. This client, conversely, would rather not burden anyone with her problems, echoing the gendered notions of endurance discussed in chapter 2. Kim described herself as initially lost with this client yet insists that she does not need to adapt the CBT techniques themselves to a Vietnamese clientele. Rather, she only modifies her approach to them. For example, Kim explicitly states the therapeutic goals to her Western clients but tries to get her Vietnamese ones to realize what those goals are on their own, because she does not want to shame them for not knowing. What gets adapted in this cross-cultural therapeutic encounter, then, is not the CBT techniques but the clients.

TEACHING PEOPLE HOW TO FEEL

Tuấn had ambitions for how psychotherapy could help people not just one-on-one, in individual therapy sessions, but through a series of programming across print and online media platforms: self-help books, a blog, and a YouTube channel. This was less of a public health measure than an entrepreneurial effort to develop a brand—perhaps even a psychotherapeutic empire. Technology transfers inspire

Tuấn's business model. For example, he tells clients that the brain is a piece of hardware that sometimes gets a virus, and he provides the software that deletes the virus. Tuấn transfers these technologies of the self through psychoeducation, the process of providing information on mental health concerns to clients and, when appropriate, their caregivers. A central component of many psychotherapies, it rests on the assumption that understanding one's emotional challenges and how to cope with them leads to greater self-efficacy. Within the global mental health movement, the promotion of psychoeducation encourages emotional self-control, stress management, and maintaining social relationships in order to foster a general sense of wellness and produce social and economic benefits (Duncan 2017; Rose 2019).

An increasingly prominent feature of psy-globalization (Duncan 2018), lists of emotions are designed to help people label and articulate them in culturally intelligible forms (Pritzker 2016; Wilce and Fenigsen 2016). For example, Kim often shows both adult and child clients an emotions reference sheet with cartoon drawings of exaggerated facial expressions. Clients are tasked with labeling the feelings depicted in each figure in order to practice, recognize, and discuss their own emotions. When Kim asks them how they felt about some event that bothers them, many often respond by saying something such as "I didn't like it," "I thought it was stupid," or "I just walked out." Indeed, in my own research, I noticed that when Ho Chi Minh City residents recount a story, they tend to describe in detail people's actions, where an American like myself might expect a description of a perceived emotional state. In the West, emotion charts are often used for clients with alexithymia, the inability to recognize and articulate emotions in the self. While people with alexithymia may experience emotions, they can only describe them in terms of physical symptoms or externalized behavior. Typically used for subclinical conditions, here the emotions reference sheet is used to "treat" Vietnamese narrative conventions because CBT is unproductive if clients are not sufficiently descriptive of their own emotions. According to Kim, people have to feel more than "bad," because "bad" is not a feeling. Clients expand their emotional vocabulary in session and at home with various "homework" assignments like thought records or diaries. Thus, clients are not taught to feel for the first time, as Vi and some of her classmates might surmise. Rather, as one of the first steps in their treatment, they learn to impose categories of emotions on their lives.

While specific emotions may be supported in some cultural contexts (e.g., anger among the Ilongot; Rosaldo 1983) but avoided in others (e.g., anger among the Inuit; Briggs 1970), cultivating an awareness and receptiveness to a broad range of emotions is increasingly valorized in neoliberalizing contexts. After all, Kim wants to teach people how to feel, not what to feel. Some refer to the general category of emotions through the term *nỗi niềm*, which is a combination of the classifier for both negative (*nỗi*, as in *nỗi buồn*, or sorrow) and positive (*niềm*, as in *niềm vui*, or joy) emotions. Such inclusive valuation of emotional range facilitates the emotional labor, flexible subjectivities, and acceptance of others' emotional reactions that are characteristic of late capitalism (Urciuoli 2008). Through the explicit use of talking about one's thoughts, feelings, and relationships, clients learn to center themselves within their own narratives (Kirmayer 2006).

Clients also learn to disentangle themselves from the rhythms of everyday life. For example, one stress management exercise is to ask people to recall the last time they were stressed. For Tuấn, that people usually cannot remember is evidence of a lack of emotional intelligence. At his stress management workshops, he asks participants how a person in Ho Chi Minh City, where just going outside entails bumping up against ten million other people, goes a single day without stress. The goal of the stress management workshops is to increase attendees' awareness of potential triggers so that they can be more conscious of their own frustrations and manage them in ways that do not harm others. Đức, a forty-five-year-old clinical psychologist at an international hospital in Ho Chi Minh City, explains the concept of "taking it out on others" to his Vietnamese clients with the expression *"giận cá chém thớt"* (so angry at the fish that you slash through the cutting board). The imposition of a medico-scientific model of psychic distress—which is to say, redrawing the line between self and society—does not necessarily flatten people's emotional lives so much as frame the everyday as an arena for emotional experience. Unlike some of his peers in Ho Chi Minh City, Tuấn believed that Vietnamese people were already too emotional. As such, they need emotional intelligence to observe their own feelings and, thus, to be more aware of and subsequently manage themselves. This particular type of self-awareness distinguishes the core of the self from the circumstances, so that one is able to separate the two.

The use of CBT to cultivate an emotive self submerged in the demands of everyday life in Vietnam may be surprising to many CBT practitioners in the United States, where one of the most popular psychotherapeutic trends of late is mindfulness-based cognitive therapy (MBCT). This modified version of CBT incorporates mindfulness meditation, which was most popularized in the West by the Vietnamese Buddhist monk Thích Nhất Hạnh. According to MBCT theory, feelings come and go and do not represent who one is, so one should not attach one's identity to how one feels at any given moment. Thus, by observing their thoughts and withholding any judgment about them, clients disengage from both everyday life and their feelings. Mindfulness-based practices are also gaining traction in Vietnam, but not just within psychotherapeutic circles. Ho Chi Minh City's corporate culture has embraced meditation in the secular pursuit of people's professional ambitions, with seemingly little attention to the Buddhist warnings about attachment and striving (Nguyen 2020).

Teaching people "how to feel" is less about the production of affective states than the cultivation of an emotive self. While CBT may reconfigure people's models of the self to align them with the rational behaviors that the state and market economy encourage, it can also provide inspiration in rethinking the relationship between self and others. Working on the self may be done to repair social relationships, not sever them (Pritzker and Duncan 2019). Participants at Tuấn's stress management workshops learn to identify and cope with stress in more productive ways. For example, Tuấn suggests going to the gym or getting a drink with friends before going home from a particularly stressful day at the office. While taking some time for oneself can be interpreted as a typically neoliberal form of self-care, in this case it is done to avoid taking the stress home, where it might create conflict. This becomes a way to renegotiate, as opposed to escape, relationships in the context of radical social transformations (Duncan 2018). Thus, the realms of the individual and the social are not necessarily in opposition to one another but instead are mutually contingent (Yates-Doerr 2015). Rather than establishing a monolithic form of selfhood, psychoeducation contributes to "meta-emotional diversity" (Wilce and Fenigsen 2016, 83). Psychotherapy has become an arena in which people can experiment with alternative and hybrid identities in the context of rapid social change.

THE POLITICIZATION OF PSYCHOLOGIZATION

Because psychotherapeutic practices frame individual interiority and autonomy as a matter of personal growth, counseling privileges clients' subjective experiences over their political-economic circumstances. As a result, therapeutic practices encourage people to mine and then manifest their inner selves to achieve their personal goals instead of questioning their sociopolitical circumstances. For example, in post-Maoist China, the state integration of psychotherapeutic measures and techniques in police, military, and labor matters renders political-economic quandaries in emotive terms (Yang 2014; Zhang 2017, 2020). Drawing on psychological expertise to understand political problems obviates the neglected and unmet responsibilities of the state by focusing on individuals for their inability to adapt to their new economic circumstances. From this perspective, psychotherapy becomes a means to induct people into the state's therapeutic ethos and to cloak its deficiencies by distracting them from growing inequalities.

While some aspects of these criticisms certainly resonate in Vietnam, psychotherapeutic discourses have also been mobilized as a form of social critique of Vietnam's political past and present. Indeed, the state of the country's mental health burden has long been viewed as an indictment against the existing social order. In the early twentieth century, Vietnam's academic, popular, and literary press became the site of intense debate over and experimentation with the role of the self in public and family life. For example, citing Émile Durkheim, Vietnamese scholars argued that rising rates of mental illness and suicide were the byproducts of modernization, not a deficiency in traditional culture (Edington 2019). Between World Wars I and II, the Vietnamese intelligentsia resisted colonial rule by drawing on Western scientific knowledge and medicine that the French believed were too advanced for Vietnamese to appreciate (Nguyễn-Võ 2008).

While mental-health-related critiques from the colonial era swirled around debates about whether or not the Vietnamese had the intellectual capacity to govern themselves, today they center on emotional maturity, specifically the development of the emotional intelligence necessary to rise to the challenges of a fast-paced market economy. Psychotherapists' assessments of the national state of feeling offer implicit critiques of the state. For example, their explanations for the current interest in emotion and mental health concerns typically attribute its emergence to social changes introduced by đổi mới–era globalization or modernization. Emotional intelligence is simultaneously understood as a universal feature of humanity and a product of the country's recent economic growth, which many Ho Chi Minh City residents attribute not to effective strategic measures on the part of the state but rather to its withdrawal from the public sphere. In Ho Chi Minh City, the ruling Communist Party is often considered an interruption not only in people's lives but also in the city's cultural and economic identity as the primary engine of Vietnam's economic growth. In this timeline of progress, the entrepreneurialism of the southern Vietnamese is a matter of instinct (Leshkowich 2014a).

Most of the blame for the current state of feeling, however, is reserved for Vietnamese neo-Confucianism because it stands for the traditions that prevent people from adopting a modern mindset. For example, Kim argued that strict parenting styles and heavy school and household workloads prevent Vietnamese teenagers from a phase of rebellious self-expression. In Vietnam's patrilocal residence pattern, individuals rarely leave their family homes until they establish a family of their own. Because most people only move from one family into another, they are too focused on pleasing others to discover how to meet their own desires. For example, Hoa and Khuyên (from chapter 2) defined their emotional maturity in terms of care, sentiment, and sacrifice. Khuyên's mother told her she was mature for her age because Khuyên never made her sad. Conversely, Kim advised a female client in her twenties who had just broken up with her boyfriend, with whom she had been cohabitating, to keep her apartment but remain single for a while so that she could learn what satisfies her.

Unlike Kim, Tuấn did not place the blame for people's emotional woes on Confucianism itself so much as on the contrast between tradition and modernity—or, as he phrased it, "rice (lúa) culture slamming up against high tech." Rapid but uneven socioeconomic transformation is testing the Vietnamese mentality. According to him, cities change at a breakneck pace, but the countryside (where most current Ho Chi Minh City residents grew up) has remained the same for the past century. It is a tumultuous time for the Vietnamese, but they do not even know it because they are distracted by the lure of modernity's shiny surfaces. This was perhaps best illustrated by a specific subject of Tuấn's ire: people with iPhones who arrive late to meetings because they got lost. According to him, they do not know how to use the maps function on their phones, which they use only to take selfies and to show off their latest status symbol. Instead of using new technologies to better their lives, people are too focused on their own vanity because they care so much about what others think of them. People are so stuck in a village mentality that they do not look beyond their immediate horizons, let alone the screens of their smartphones. Tuấn also blamed Buddhist notions of fate (số mệnh) for encouraging passivity and preventing people from taking responsibility for their own actions. "Good luck taking on scientific values," he said, "because that is the future."

Thus, when CBT practitioners describe the challenges of providing care in Vietnam, they are careful not to blame their clients for some deficiency of individuality or personal responsibility, among others. Instead, the blame gets shifted onto Vietnamese culture and politics. CBT's intense focus on the inner self often comes at the expense of social and cultural factors that restrict people's ability to implement changes for themselves. Any factors stemming from so-called cultural traditions that deviate from CBT's presumed ideal of personhood are presented as detrimental or even as quasi-pathological or pathogenic. Psychotherapists link the nation's changing tides with the minds of its citizens, and many of them stated that psychology is the most important field for the country's future. In their argument, addressing Vietnam's mental health crisis is essential to modernizing the country, as if "modernity" and its trappings were not part of the problem to begin with.

CONCLUSION

Taken together, pharmaceutical and psychotherapeutic treatments for anxiety reveal the breadth of ways in which selfhood has been adapted to meet people's needs in post-reform Vietnam. Because pharmaceutical approaches in Vietnam directly focus on the physical symptoms of anxiety, patients are largely able to accommodate them into their existing understandings of worry, illness, and selfhood. Doctors' entreaties to reexamine patients' personal lives, if even bothered with, went largely ignored. Psychotherapeutic treatments, conversely, target and challenge clients' sense of self, not just their symptoms. Almost in spite of itself, CBT has become a critical means of self-discovery in Vietnam. If, as I have argued, models of selfhood are inextricable from different forms of anxiety, new configurations of the self—even those designed to ease troubled minds—may elicit different forms of anxiety. Ho Chi Minh City residents seeking relief from their worries may get more than they bargained for in their sessions.

"What's the difference between psychology and anthropology?" Trâm asked me. She apologized for still being unclear about my profession even after years of friendship, but she could hardly be blamed. Psychotherapy sessions and the person-centered ethnographic interviews that Trâm had participated in share common attributes, including an exploration of the significance of one's feelings, relative anonymity—at least from the clients and interviewees' social networks— and the mutual construction of empathy.[6] However, as I told Trâm, anthropological research typically does not have the therapeutic goal of changing people's behavior. Instead, it aims to contextualize their experiences in political and economic institutions. At any rate, I knew her well enough to know that her next question—"You studied psychology in school, right?"—had an ulterior motive. Trâm suggested that she could tell her story (kể chuyện) and I could then explain her own psyche to her. I insisted that I was no substitute for a therapist but could listen as a friend. I also offered to put her in contact with some of the psychotherapists I knew, but she said she could not afford it anyway. Her proposal reflects both the growing interest in psychotherapy throughout Ho Chi Minh City and how out-of-reach it is for many. Regardless, Trâm had long experimented, to varying degrees of success, with the emotive discourses of the self that Ho Chi Minh City's mental health workers promote. The next chapter examines some of these attempts, from several years prior to this conversation, and how psychotherapeutic ideals of emotion and selfhood operate outside of the clinic.

PART THREE

Anxious Formations

6

Love, Anxiety

INTO THE WILD

Shortly after graduating from Emory University with bachelor's degrees in history and anthropology in 1990, Christopher Johnson McCandless sold most of his possessions and, under the pseudonym Alexander Supertramp, worked odd jobs across the United States. His two years on the road, a testament to self-reliance, self-discovery, and romanticized individualism, culminated in a Jack London–esque "Alaskan odyssey." Stranded, lost, and alone for four months in Denali National Park, McCandless died of starvation, and it remains open to interpretation whether his death was accidental or suicidal in nature. A shrine built where he died became a destination for many adventurers fascinated by his story, which was first popularized by the book *Into the Wild* by Jon Krakauer (1996).

Eighteen-year-old Thịnh saw the film adaptation of *Into the Wild* (Penn 2007) and often talked about it with an American woman,[1] ten years his senior, who was a regular customer at his parents' small drinking establishment in the foothills of the Central Highlands. He developed a habit of sending her ponderous text messages, which she either only politely responded to or ignored. Late one night, he arrived unannounced at the house she was renting a room in to announce his devotion to her. When he asked her if she loved him, she firmly said "Không" (No) and told him to go home. Thịnh did but continued to send text messages nearly nonstop, eventually writing that her personal happiness was more important to him than her reciprocating his feelings. Because of this, he would stop all contact with her if she wished. She did not respond to any of these messages. Around 3:00 a.m. he texted to announce that this was to be his last communication with her because he was going to go "into the wild." He snuck one of his parents' motorbikes out of the house and drove eight hours to his sister's apartment in Ho Chi Minh City.

105

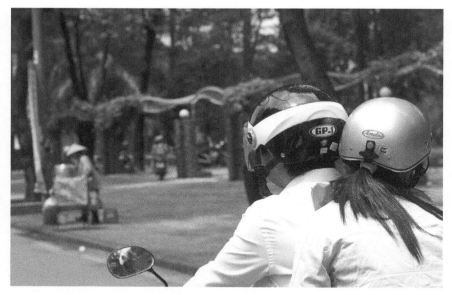

FIGURE 5. Motorbikes and urban anonymity have made romantic intimacy possible in the public sphere, especially in Ho Chi Minh City's downtown.

WINDS OF CHANGE

The first time she drove a motorbike, Trâm crashed into a vegetable stand. Now in her mid-thirties, she often told this story from her adolescence in Ho Chi Minh City to prove her occasional reckless streak. Young Vietnamese women are supposed to be gentle (*hiền*), but Trâm described herself as fierce (*dữ*). While she acknowledged that she had mellowed with age, I still found her to be unusually direct, and she clearly reveled in telling me when I made a mistake. For example, meeting her at a different café than our usual lunch spot, I misused the Vietnamese idiom "a change of wind" (*đổi gió*), which I assumed was equivalent to the expression "a change of scenery." Trâm cracked a smile as she informed me that "a change of wind" is reserved for more dramatic changes than trying a new restaurant.

Sometimes, Trâm continued, she daydreamed about going by herself to Vũng Tàu, a coastal city two and a half hours away by motorbike from Ho Chi Minh City. This struck me as odd for two reasons. First, the idea of wanting to go on an excursion by oneself, or even wanting more than a few hours of alone time, was relatively uncommon in Vietnam at the time.[2] Second, the tone of our typical banter quietly turned serious. What was Trâm trying to escape? Why would someone as forthright and pragmatic as her take such drastic action to avoid confrontation? Would she ever act on it, or was just the thought enough for her?

I was unaware of it at the time, but the subtext of Trâm's fantasy was crisis: the recent discovery of her husband's extramarital affair. For months afterward, she and her husband bickered constantly over trivial matters, and it seemed that the only times they were not arguing were when they were not speaking to each other at all. Trâm came home one afternoon only to have her husband harangue her over some unwashed dishes before she could put down her keys. She turned on her heels, walked downstairs to the apartment building's parking garage, and drove to Vũng Tàu.[3]

IN AND OUT OF LOVE

What do Ho Chi Minh City residents worry about as they fall in and out of love? To answer this question, we must situate the interpersonal experiences of romantic love and emotional intimacy in their sociopolitical context. Emerging forms of romance in Vietnam promote a reorientation of the self toward the love object in a manner that affirms modernist fantasies of intimate recognition. When middle-class Ho Chi Minh City residents discuss love, which they often do, they speak specifically about the objects of their affection, their intentions, and their plans. In doing so, they affirm a contemporary vision of their love lives that is convention-alized as entailing the mutual recognition of—and resulting intimacy between—two individuals (Berlant 2012). However, new romantic formations do not simply replace Confucian and socialist ideals of affection that prioritize collective obliga-tions. Rather, they reconfigure them into a hybrid of conflicting models of modern selfhood in Vietnam. The ways that Vietnamese draw from and invest in romantic tropes of selfhood to fashion themselves as modern subjects vary from person to person, but two problems are consistent: determining the authenticity of romantic love and reconciling the gap between the objects of people's affections and what gets projected onto those objects (Berlant 2012).

While many of my respondents believe that following their hearts instead of obliging filial duty or Confucian gender roles makes them "modern," I contend that their relation to modernity is not only defined by intimacy and the acknowl-edgment of their individuality. The anxieties of the self that romantic self-mak-ing projects inspire and are contingent upon are equally, if not more, critical to modernist identities and selfhood. According to Salecl (2020), love anxiety arises from the experiences of one's own self as undermined yet expanded and redefined through romantic entanglements. Not only does anxiety reveal the contours and effects of romance as a political self-making project, it is critical to the experience of romantic love itself. For Ho Chi Minh City's middle class, love and anxiety do not just coincide with but co-animate each other.

To demonstrate the intersection of romance, anxiety, and socioeconomic trans-formation, this chapter presents two case studies, that of Trâm and that of Hải, a twenty-year-old man who, like Thịnh, developed unrequited feelings for a West-ern woman. The betrayed wife and the unrequited lover were two of the most common figures in the stories about the agonies of romantic love recounted to me throughout my fieldwork. Together, they disclose several key factors that shape the romantic trajectories of Ho Chi Minh City residents attempting to form romantic relationships based on "both the grammar of love and the grammar of the market" (Nguyen 2007, 287), including how Confucianism and socialism are marshalled in the process. However, Trâm's and Hải's experiences are not meant to be representative of romantic relationships in Vietnam, let alone in Ho Chi Minh City. They do not reflect the complexities of increasingly visible same-sex relationships or even more conventionally successful couples, and their versions of romance reflect their age, gender, and class differences. Hải grew up under đổi mới and embraced its effects. Attending English courses and frequenting expat bars, he used his family's financial resources to self-consciously craft a hybrid Vietnamese-Western identity. Conversely, older and less economically secure than Hải, Trâm held more conservative attitudes about đổi mới and regularly framed her decisions to me in terms of traditional gender norms, even as she frequently flouted them. Although Trâm and Hải are invested in the same romantic discourses, how they interpret and enact them reflects the relation between their particular subject positions and modernity itself.

Ethnographic case studies of people rejecting, adapting, and internalizing conflicting discourses of love and late modernity indicate that if, indeed, romance is a modernizing self-making project, it is not a teleological undertaking (Zigon 2013; Davis 2014). Emphasizing individuals' romantic experiences challenges overgeneralizing claims about gender or class ideologies by attending to the dynamic process of how global trends are incorporated (or not) into people's sense of self. In Vietnam, romantic formations associated with neoliberalism are interpreted through and made possible by Confucian and socialist models of selfhood. Focusing on case studies not only reveals convergences and contradictions among the various models of romance and selfhood but also between individuals and their social milieu as they attempt to balance being in love with social obligation.[4]

While I conducted person-centered ethnographic interviews on many topics with Trâm and Hải and observed them in numerous settings, this chapter draws mainly from conversations about their romantic predicaments.[5] These exchanges occurred over a span of several months, usually at cafés and restaurants but sometimes at mutual friends' homes, where I observed how their friends and relatives reacted to their troubles.[6] I do not attempt to determine the truth of Trâm's and Hải's feelings; I leave them to struggle with those questions themselves. While the stories and perspectives they offered during our conversations do not give direct access to their inner selves, they do reveal the general understandings of selfhood, gender, and emotion that Trâm and Hải draw upon to interpret their experiences. Thus, I focus on their attempts to articulate and rework these implicit models to achieve their own goals. The analysis of both case studies was guided by four basic questions. First, what are the primary and secondary attachments for the subjects? That is, who or what is the love object, and what possibilities do the objects suggest? Second, what are the institutional norms that produce such attachments?

Third, how can the subjects of the case studies attain their goals, or what can they do to close the gap between themselves and the object of their affections? Finally, how do the subjects reencounter themselves in this process?

Both Trâm and Hải shared their dilemmas with me not simply because we were, and remain, friends but because, as an anthropologist, I mostly listened. Echoing many psychotherapists' critiques of styles of emotional support, their other friends too often gave unsolicited advice and did not—perhaps could not—understand them the way they wanted to be recognized. Hải's ardor was dismissed as irrational, and Trâm in particular worried that others would criticize her and did not want to invite public judgment on the state of her marriage. This is not to imply that I understood them better than their loved ones. However, by allowing them to explore their feelings without opining on them, I attempted to do so differently than many of their friends and family, and perhaps this was enough.

Neither Trâm nor Hải expressed any interest in consulting a psychotherapist for their issues, but both sometimes asked me for advice as if I were one. To this, I told them it was not my place to do so. Moreover, they also wanted my perspective as a foreigner on romantic love, which they imagined to be a universal experience yet one increasingly shaped in Vietnam by Western expectations of gender, emotion, and choice. As events unfolded, I became not just a witness to their romantic problems but a coconspirator in plans to resolve them. Indeed, Trâm's and Hải's interactions with me likely shaped the insights they gained about their own situations over time as my interview questions prompted them to reconsider their assumptions about love, themselves, and Vietnamese culture, among others. This chapter explores the possibilities—romantic and otherwise—that the objects of Trâm's and Hải's affections give rise to, and the social norms that create these attachments. Furthermore, following Berlant (2012), I examine what they do in order to close the gap between themselves and the objects of their affections, and how they reencounter themselves in the process.

THE THEORETICAL IMPORTANCE OF LOVE

Ethnographic scholarship on the politics of romantic love focuses on the different tactics that people use to navigate new forms of emotional and sexual intimacy and highlights the ways in which emotion and social action become fused as simultaneously tacit and culturally elaborated, embodied and rational, and spoken and unspoken (Rebhun 1999; Ahearn 2001; Hirsch and Wardlow 2006; Yan 2003; Padilla et al. 2008; Cole 2010; Zigon 2013; Nelson and Jankowiak 2021).[7] Love has been further theorized in relation to global capitalism, discourses of emotion, and political technologies of population control (Collier 1997; Freeman 2007; Friedman 2005; Hirsch and Wardlow 2006; Lipset 2004; Ryang 2006; Davis 2014). Romance has long been an arena for the struggles and experiments in freedom, choice, and self-making connected to the rise of a modernist identity defined as an individuated self with unique traits.[8] While premodern contractual marriages were based more on financial considerations than on sexual attraction, modern romantic marriages feature an emotional intimacy that is predicated on individuals' characters fulfilling each others' mutually incomplete selves (Giddens 1993; Cherlin 2004). With the increased mobility, competition, and individualism associated with capitalism, people sought refuge from the new uncertainties of the marketplace in marriage. However, romance was not simply extricated from economic contingencies in the modern era. It has assumed many of modernity's hallmarks, including rationalization, disenchantment, and a therapeutic discourse of the self (Illouz 2012). Love has become more than duty; it is the outcome of individual desires and a romantic endeavor that supports psychological and existential security. Economic transformations produce new forms and understandings of desire, which in turn create different ways of relating to others (Stout 2014; Wilson 2004).

Economic transformations produce new forms of desire and different ways of relating to others (Povinelli 2006). The emotional intimacy that characterizes modern romance depends on the self-reflexive ability to articulate one's feelings to oneself and one's romantic partners. Under neoliberalism, marriages based on affective relationships instead of external institutions produce anxiety because individuals bear responsibility for their own happiness (Illouz 1997). Moreover, within the structure of contemporary forms of romantic love, there is, perhaps more often than not, a gap between the object of one's affection and the possibilities generated by one's desires projected onto the love object (Berlant 2012). Thus, romantic love connects emergent notions of individual freedom and self-realization by provoking self-interrogation: how do I feel about the love object, and how does the love object feel about me (Lindholm 1998)? The ethnographic material that this article draws from is permeated by the question of whether or not another's love is real. This question is simultaneously psychological and political: psychological because it concerns the veracity of emotional knowledge, and political because it entails how investments in fulfilling certain fantasies are produced by social institutions (Povinelli 2006; Berlant 2012).

Love is one of the most influential modernist projects of the self, but it is one that demands others to validate one's emotion work (Illouz 2012). Intersubjectivity is not merely the merger of isolated subjects, because encounters with others cannot be reduced to a mere emanation of the constitutive subject (Crossley 1996; Csordas 2008). Emotions do not merely happen to people but are instead social actions that shape the boundaries between the individual and the social that allow them to be made known to each other (Jenkins 1994). Thus, love strains the integrity of the self so that "self and society are faced with each other" (Ryang 2006, 1; Throop 2010a; Zigon 2013). The ethnographic material that this chapter draws from is permeated by the question of whether someone's love is real.

Though typically described in vaunted and heady terms, love can be just as anxiety-inducing. That anxiety and love are as conceptually differentiated as they often are is a curious matter, since many of the same expressions used to describe their respective phenomenological experiences refer to a common set of physical states that include heightened arousal, internal feelings of flux, and sensations exceeding the limits of the body. Vulnerability, insecurity, and uncertainty often characterize romance, in effect acknowledging the importance of the love object to a person and that person's need and lack of control over the love object (Nussbaum 2001). While anxiety notably does not have an object (May 1950), romantic love is distinct because the object is often so vivid. When else do we have a more intimate sense of the object? A step toward a more rigorous examination of how love and anxiety are related to each other could be to demarcate their boundaries. However, doing so reifies static categories. Instead, I focus on the interpenetration of what gets labeled as anxiety and/or romantic love and how they are coproduced by political-economic transformations.

VIETNAM'S ROMANTIC HISTORY

French literature introduced Western notions of romance (*lãng mạn*) and love (*tình yêu*) into Vietnam during the colonial period (1887–1954). Popular with urban youth in the 1930s, the *Thơ Mới* (New Poetry) and *Tự Lực Văn Đoàn* (Self-Reliance Literary Group) movements examined conflicts between romance and filial duty and the cultivation of emotionality, especially love, for the sake of modernizing (Phinney 2008a). The incorporation of new literary conventions into Vietnamese poetry and fiction incubated new concepts of the individual that would facilitate the spread of socialism in northern Vietnam (McHale 1995; Marr 2000). However, romance was delegitimized by socialist modernity as public affect was directed toward the state and loyalties outside of the individual and the state, including family obligations, were discouraged (Schwenkel 2013). The International Communist Party, in particular, exhorted youth to be nation builders as vanguards of the socialist revolution. Women were encouraged to join the Party as a way to liberate themselves from the patriarchal confines of the family (Tai 1992). Young wives upset that their husbands were sent to war were chastised for being selfish, bourgeois, and Western and encouraged to redefine love as a sacrifice to the nation (Pettus 2003).

Romance in Vietnam has long been an acceptable condition for courtship, but people have only more recently come to expect it in marriage. In Ho Chi Minh City, young people are often concerned with finding a romantic partner who will fulfill customary marital roles (e.g., male breadwinners and female caretakers), much like their parents and grandparents. However, they also increasingly prioritize receiving emotional satisfaction and self-fulfillment from their partners. One of the ways in which Ho Chi Minh City residents realize a "modern" identity is by drawing from romantic idioms of the self as individuals in search of romantic partners uniquely suited to them instead of having marriages arranged for them (Hirschman and Nguyen 2002; Earl 2014a).[9] State-envisioned subjectivity in the reform era shifted from "revolutionary love" and "socialist love" in emphases on the individual's allegiance to the state to one of a happy, healthy, and wealthy family. The shift from building the nation to focusing on one's family is necessary for the creation of citizens responsible for themselves and the nation's rise in the global economy (Phinney 2008a). In effect, the state yielded its position as an object of sentiment and love once the household was established as the primary economic unit (Nguyễn-Võ 2008); conjugal and family love replaced it. Instead of being a haven from the vagaries of the marketplace, "modern romantic love is a practice intimately complicit with the political economy of capitalism" (Illouz 1997, 22).

Today, popular discourses about romantic love (*tình yêu*) within and beyond Vietnam often assume its universality, with the result that it gets placed on a spiritual pedestal as proof of our shared humanity. In its purest distillations, love should be independent of financial and material vagaries, even overcoming them if need be. For example, Thuận (from chapter 2) told me that he had "cried like a baby" when his girlfriend Vy (from chapter 3) broke up with him. Because of her family's limited economic means, her parents insisted that she marry an over- seas Vietnamese man so that she could move to the West and secure their future through economic remittances (Small 2018). Thuận interpreted her acquiescence not just as her not loving him enough to defy her parents, but as their relationship having never been based on "true love"[10] at all. (Now working in the marketing department at a multinational corporation, Thuận owns a house and car. He and his new wife went on a lavish honeymoon in Paris.) The ways that Vietnamese draw from and invest in romantic tropes of the self to fashion themselves as mod- ern subjects vary from person to person, but what is consistent are the problems of determining the authenticity of romantic love and the gap between the objects of people's affections and all that is projected onto them. That is, within the struc- ture of contemporary forms of romantic love, there is, perhaps more often than not, a gap between the object of one's affection and the possibilities generated by one's desires projected onto the love object (Berlant 2012). Romantic love connects emergent notions of individual freedom and self-realization by provoking self- interrogation: how do I feel about the love object, and how does the love object feel about me (Lindholm 1998)?

TRÂM

If Love

Trâm and Danh had been married for nearly ten years without much incident, which was part of the problem. Unable to conceive a child, the couple consulted biomedical fertility specialists and fortune tellers alike, spending vast sums of money on hormone therapy medication and votive goods to burn at auspicious temples. Meanwhile, Danh seemed to regress into bachelorhood, spending more time and money with his friends than with Trâm. Like many of her female friends, Trâm fondly recalled Danh's chivalrous gestures during their courtship, but these memories now served to remind her of how much had since changed. Throughout Vietnam, wives desire intimacy and perform more emotional labor than their husbands (Vu 2020). Before they were married, Trâm's passing mention of a headache over the phone to Danh would occasion an unexpected delivery of aspirin to her office during his lunch break. Now, she went to the pharmacy by herself—for much bigger headaches, she insisted—even after asking him to go for her.

The state of Trâm's marriage was defined by three interrelated dissatisfactions that reflected her own fraught relationship with modernity. First was the problem of a stalled rise into the middle class. Although generally supportive of đổi mới, Trâm criticized many of its social consequences, including the sexual openness of urban youth and the increasing anonymity in her once tightly knit neighborhood. Moreover, as peers with more financial resources and personal connections attained what many Vietnamese consider to be modern lifestyles, she felt excluded from đổi mới's economic effects and found herself on the fringes of Ho Chi Minh City's upwardly mobile. Trâm admitted to me that she was envious of her best friend, Vân-Anh, watching as she got married, gave birth, and bought a house and eventually a car. Meanwhile, Trâm and Danh had been living in her domineering mother's apartment since they got married. (The Vietnamese postmarital residence pattern is patrilocal, but Trâm refused to live with her spendthrift in-laws.) According to Trâm, her living situation reflected both the uneven distribution of đổi mới's benefits and Danh's inability to provide her with a "good life."

The various markers of the Vietnamese middle class and modernity itself promise a greater degree of personal autonomy, especially for women. Criticizing patriarchal Confucianism as feudal, she and many others I knew in Ho Chi Minh City believe—despite my repeated protestations otherwise—that Western men and women are enlightened equals who choose for themselves how to be emotionally fulfilled. Regardless, what Trâm considered modern, anchored in an idealization of gender and freedom, shaped the horizon of her romantic aspirations. Given that she imagined middle-class modernity in terms of personal freedom, it is no surprise that romance was critical to her own happiness.

Second, the inability to conceive a child both created immense personal turmoil for Trâm and underscored the effects of Vietnam's political-economic transitions. Although marriage in Vietnam reflects Confucian, socialist, and neoliberal configurations, the dominant marital discourse emphasizes a set of customary roles delineated by Confucianism (Goodkind 1996; Soucy 2001). Since the principal function of Confucian and socialist models of marriage is, respectively, continuing the patrilineage and boosting population quality (Pashigian 2009; Gammeltoft 2014a), what justifications remained for Trâm and Danh's relationship? How else could they meet each other's needs—if they even needed each other anymore? While Vietnam has an established tradition of spousal obligations (tình nghĩa) that may or may not be accompanied by feelings of love, it is based on a social order that has recently become less salient for urban youth. Trâm often said that in courtship, love is destined (*duyên*) to happen or not; in marriage, love is owed. She believed that raising a child together and focusing on a shared goal would bring her and Danh closer as a familial unit.

Third, the absence of a child to focus Trâm and Danh's attention allowed them to drift apart, highlighting the unfulfilling romance of their marriage. While Danh had no "knack for observation," Trâm was keenly aware of her husband's habits, preferences, and schedules but felt increasingly estranged from his thoughts. Perhaps the greatest attraction of romantic marriage for Trâm and her friends lay in the emphasis on intimacy as a matter of emotional communication and interpersonal equality. Intimacy and the democratization of men and women in the private sphere are based on recognition of the other's individual characteristics (Giddens 1993). While a desire for emotional intimacy between spouses is not solely rooted in modernist configurations of selfhood and marriage, it takes on the form of what Trâm imagined to be Western expectations of emotional expressiveness.

Shaped by neoliberal conventions of emotional intimacy and Confucian expectations of gendered obligation, Trâm's desires led to an impasse. She wanted a marriage based on romantic ideals but was unsure how to propagate one without a child to draw her and Danh closer. For example, asked to describe how their initial romance could be revived, Trâm explained that Danh needs to take better care of her by taking her out more often and buying their own home. That is, she answered in terms of fulfilling Confucian socioeconomic roles. Trâm's idealization of Western romance overlooked the emphasis on the recognition and communication of one's feelings that characterizes neoliberal formations of marriage (Illouz 2012). Indeed, she seemed to me unaware of even holding competing models of marriage. Rarely mentioning her own faults in her marriage's problems in our conversations, Trâm effectively refused to participate in the reflexive self-making project of modern romance. Whether this was due to inertia or resistance to neoliberal ideals of selfhood mattered little, as a crisis would compel her to take one up.

Outside of Love

Ly had recently left her husband, not realizing that her in-laws would prevent any contact with her three-year-old son. She confided in Danh, whom she met through his work as a sales representative, and they eventually became friends. Trâm described feeling a sympathetic twinge in her stomach when Danh explained Ly's plight to her. However, Danh went on to confess that his initial feelings of compassion toward Ly had turned into attraction.[11] He insisted that he did not have any sexual contact with her and affirmed his loyalty to Trâm, promising to discontinue his friendship with Ly. Not wanting to stand between two people who loved each other, Trâm even went to Ly's house to yield (*nhường*) Danh to her. Ly asked Trâm if she was crazy.

It was a few weeks later, late at night, when Trâm was next in the neighborhood, this time to deliver a gift to a friend who coincidentally lived a few houses from Ly. The dim light and shadows made it difficult for Trâm to make out the two familiar silhouettes not too far from her. The man leaning against a motorbike, they stood next to one another—not so close as to warrant much attention from passersby, but close enough to disclose an intimacy. When Trâm called out her husband's name, the couple turned toward her, faces still obscured in the shadows, but their attention was confirmation enough. She immediately went to her in-laws' home to report Danh's infidelity. She asked her father-in-law three times to take his son back, but he refused. That night, Danh returned home to her, which she took as a sign that he still loved her.

Trâm drew from various models of marriage, emotion, and selfhood to determine the authenticity of love, both hers and his. The most clearly articulated account of Danh's betrayal related to domains such as spousal responsibilities and finances that resonate with dominant discourses of infidelity (*ngoại tình*, lit. outside love). Marital infidelity has become a flashpoint for conflicting opinions about *đổi mới* (Horton and Rydstrom 2011). High rates of adultery are regarded as extensions of a feudal tradition of polygyny.[12] Many blame the corrupting influence of the West for purveying sexual libertinism and immoral lifestyles that people succumb to. Rapid urbanization and an increase in disposable income provide anonymity and an availability of sexual partners and have intensified the commercial significance of the sex work industry (Hoang 2015; Nguyễn-Võ 2008).[13] Unfaithful husbands are faulted for their weakness and irresponsibility in jeopardizing stable families. The women involved are positioned against one another vis-à-vis husbands: wives as morally pure, passive victims expected to forgive their husbands and extramarital partners as greedy and manipulative temptresses. Such is the power of these competing discourses that Trâm claimed Ly did not truly love Danh and only wanted his money, despite Trâm's repeated complaints that he had none.

However, the more pressing accounts of Trâm's betrayal—the ones that seemed to bother her more because she had not yet come to terms with them—focused on Danh's emotional dishonesty.[14] She could produce a list of things that Danh could do to take better care of her but did not know what he could do to restore trust and intimacy to their relationship. That is, she had greater difficulty articulating the violation and resolution of a model of marriage as an emotional institution. Indeed, she was not sure if she could trust Danh again or even if he had stopped seeing Ly. Over the following months, Trâm made several attempts to identify the affective roots of her marital problems. The process of doing so not only revealed how she deployed and reconfigured assumptions about modernity, marriage, and love but also constituted her own attempted self-making project.

This endeavor to remake the self was marked by a liminality stemming from uncertainties over love's authenticity: did Trâm still love Danh, and vice versa? Modernist articulations of romantic love encourage private reflection and emotional communication to answer such questions (Illouz 2012). Trâm, however, sought to determine the authenticity of love through a series of concrete plans. According to her, whether or not these plans succeeded (i.e., whether or not she had the resolve to pull them off) would reflect her true feelings about Danh. Their purpose seemed to be less about the viability of realizing her goals than about helping her determine what those goals were. In doing so, she explored possibilities in remaking her self according to the demands of each plan.

Trâm's first plan—to divorce Danh—was perhaps her most straightforward. The drawbacks to divorce (e.g., neighborhood gossip) would be temporary, and she would be free of her in-laws. Yet she hesitated to initiate legal proceedings because staying married was the path of least resistance. Her indecisiveness also stemmed from uncertainties about what to do in her everyday interactions with Danh, which she said was the most difficult thing to bear. Trâm knew how to behave with friends or colleagues but could not accept any of the cultural scripts for dealing with her husband (i.e., either forgiving or leaving him). Her subsequent plans called for more drastic self-transformations. For example, she wanted to marry an American partly because she believed that American men routinely made romantic gestures (e.g., bringing their wives flowers), despite my repeated protestations. In her experience, Vietnamese men change after marriage and are not committed to the romantic foundations of marriage that she idealized. She enviously compared the relative sexual freedom and gender equity that she assumed American women enjoyed to the patriarchal confines that their Vietnamese counterparts endured.

Trâm knew she had only a vague understanding of what her new life in America might be like—only that it would be better than her current one in Vietnam. She worried about not being able to become someone who was attractive to or compatible with an American or, if all went well, not being able to become an American herself. That is, she worried that she did not know how to remake herself. Regardless, the possibility of the transformative properties of love—her own utopia of gender, sex, and affective life—outweighed the risks of marrying a foreigner and moving away from her family. Such fantasies of the West allowed Trâm to imagine the possibilities of her own selfhood (Parish 2008) yet also created anxieties about the gap between what she already possessed and did not yet possess. Forays into international online dating, with some assistance from Vân-Anh's better English skills, quickly dimmed Trâm's hopes. Over the next few months, she developed more schemes that she could not settle on, including one that entailed her getting pregnant but divorcing Danh soon afterward.

The back-and-forth nature of Trâm's plans suggests that she was trying to determine what to do on the basis of whether she still loved Danh, whether he still loved her, and whether they both actually loved each other—questions she had no answer to, despite how often she returned to them. I suspect that she tried to answer the question "Do I still love him?" by resolving the question of "What should I do?" That is, romantic love would follow suit from the new horizons of possibilities that she would engineer with her plans. The actualization of these possibilities was always mediated by an attachment to an Other: her current husband, her next one, or an unborn child.

Uninterested in the neoliberal imperative toward self-sufficiency, Trâm viewed romance as a vehicle toward care according to Confucian-inflected gender roles. Yet she also wanted to attain the affective intimacy and modernist ideals of emotional fulfillment that characterize romantic marriage. Throughout this period, Trâm also tried to salvage her marriage by opening a dialogue about the relationship with Danh, who refused to engage in these conversations. The suggestions she received from Vân-Anh (e.g., keeping silent when angry to avoid arguments) did little to improve the situation. I contend, however, that what hindered these conversations even more was Trâm and Danh's unfamiliarity with the self-reflexive communication about their feelings that characterizes both modern romance and identities. For many members of Ho Chi Minh City's middle class, the construction and performance of an emotive self has become critical to naturalizing neoliberal reforms (Tran 2015). Within the therapeutic discourses of the self that have become popular throughout the region, intrapersonal issues are framed as an underlying cause of interpersonal conflicts (Yang 2014), and interior contemplation should precede the more concrete courses of action that Trâm preferred. However, during our conversations, she struggled with articulating her feelings. Her romantic goals were used to guide her toward her aspirations for a middle-class life with more economic security and emotional satisfaction. However, she did not internalize a regime of the self marked by self-sufficiency or self-reflexivity, perhaps because that regime was out of her reach.

Fight and Flight

The highway to Vũng Tàu is not especially perilous, and Trâm knew it well. She was not even that angry when she left without telling anyone. Yet anxiety dominated her recall of the events. Worries about skidding off the road with no one to help her occupied her thoughts during the entire trip. She wanted to turn around, but she finally had a plan that she could actually implement by herself. Testing Danh's commitment to her, Trâm wanted to see if he would meet her in Vũng Tàu, where they could spend of the rest of the weekend to rekindle their marriage. According to her, a husband who truly loves his wife would save her from a dangerous situation, even if she had put herself in that situation. Instead, they only ended up fighting over the phone, and she spent the night in a hotel room watching TV, kept awake by unfamiliar noises she thought might be ghosts. Still, she had no regrets.

When Trâm first told me of escaping to the beach by herself, I assumed it was a way to avoid confrontation. However, it was designed to provoke one. What started out as a romantic project to transform her and Danh's intersubjective entanglements became, in the end, a solitary self-making endeavor. Trâm enjoyed challenging herself in manageable increments. By stepping out of her everyday for a mission that was different from what she (or we) expected, she discovered that she was—or made herself—bold enough to embark on new courses of action. This was a journey that she needed to make for reasons I am still unclear about, but she found out that her husband was someone who could not make it with her.

For a few months, I had minimal contact with Trâm, only seeing her with our mutual friends. When we finally had lunch again, I asked her if there was anything new in her life. Staring into her coffee, she told me about a new lover, a colleague who seemed diametrically opposed to Danh in many ways, except that they were both married. Some nights, they would sit side-by-side in the darkest corners of the café where we were then meeting. Days were romantic too. If he knew Trâm skipped lunch, he would treat the entire office to steamed pork buns for an afternoon snack. She asked me if I was surprised that she was having an affair. I said yes, but mainly insofar as she had told me multiple times she was through with men. She surprised herself as well, having become a figure that she despised. Although she believed she had every right to conduct an affair of her own, she soon ended the relationship out of guilt toward her colleague's wife and young daughter.

Many have made note of the mysticism often tied up with romance. People frequently joked to me of the love charms, tonics, and amulets used on unwitting souls, or of soothsayers consulted to divine answers to romantic uncertainties. The implication of these stories is that individual destinies are bound to broader circumstances. Certainly, Trâm had moments when she believed that her circumstances were ordained by powers far outside of her control: her husband's actions, Confucian patriarchy, or her own karma. At other times—more often than not, I would gather—she looked to a more open-ended future. Trying to balance being in love with duty and obligation, she lacked the social and economic capital (e.g., English skills, self-reflexive emotionality) necessary to successfully navigate conflicting models of romance and selfhood. For many in contemporary Vietnam, romance is no longer the stuff of fairy tales and far-flung destinies. It has turned into a realm in which individuals can seal their own fates. For Trâm, however, this did not make romance seem any less fictional.

HẢI

In Love

Whereas Trâm's romantic struggles were focused on uncertainties about the authenticity of love, in the next case study, love itself is seldom in doubt. The numerous narratives about unrequited love (*tình đơn phương*, or love in a lonely direction) I heard during fieldwork typically involved young men making grand gestures to the objects of their affection, despite repeated rejections. Enamored of the modern West as portrayed in global pop culture, Hải set out to reinvent himself when he left his hometown of Phan Thiết for college.[15] While his classmates at the University of Economics aimed for well-paying jobs upon graduation and generally snubbed him for being an unserious student, his primary goal for "studying" in Ho Chi Minh City entailed becoming modern. His version of a modern individual, however, had less to do with the consumerist lifestyles that his peers desired than with self-determination and understanding. Hải sought an alternate education found in Ho Chi Minh City's cosmopolitanism and the encounters with people and practices from the West to discover global modernity. He admitted to me, however, that his busy social calendar had the additional function of masking an underlying loneliness. Sometimes, spending time with friends, especially if they were coupled with one another, exacerbated his sense of isolation.

Hải spent three years unsuccessfully wooing Ngọc, a high school classmate who went to a different university in Ho Chi Minh City. He made up excuses to go to the apartment she shared with friends in the hopes of running into her because, according to him, he missed her and cared for her well-being. "To miss" and "to remember" are synonyms in Vietnamese (*nhớ*), and Hải was constantly reminded of Ngọc by tangential resemblances (e.g., the length of someone's hair) and would talk about his lovesickness (*thất tình*) to anybody who would listen. Quick-witted and handsome, Hải had little difficulty attracting women but usually ended those fledgling relationships after a few weeks out of loyalty to Ngọc or, it often seemed, a devotion to his own misery. Hải's friends told him to forget her, though the only advice they ever offered was to busy himself with schoolwork to appease his parents. Nobody, not even Ngọc herself, could deter him when she posted this on his social media account: "*Tôi mãi mãi sẽ không thích anh*" (I will not like you forever).

The Loneliest Direction

Hải's English teacher invited several friends for a pub crawl to covertly introduce Hải to an Australian colleague's daughter, named Abby.[16] Several drinks later, Hải and Abby were making out on an otherwise empty dance floor of a gay bar for thirty minutes in full view of everyone, including Abby's mother. Despite his aimless life, for that night, he said, "*cuộc sống là màu hồng*" (life is pink). Despite the evident elation when I met him for coffee the next morning, he was worried. Did Abby love him back? Was she only interested in sex? Would they even have sex? If they fell in love too fast, would they break up too soon? Most urgently, what happens next? Hải's subsequent interactions with Abby and their mutual friends at various venues popular with Ho Chi Minh City's English teachers were stilted, and it became clear to everyone but Hải that she did not reciprocate his feelings.

Like Trâm, Hải set out to become the type of person he hoped Westerners would find attractive. Because he barely knew Abby (something that seemed lost on him), he mostly relied on stereotypes of the West. Hải's belief that Westerners are more direct and emotional than the Vietnamese resulted in a series of increasingly desperate overtures to win Abby over. His ideas about the art of seduction were reinforced by Western pop culture but missed cultural conventions about maintaining distance that are violated for entertainment purposes. For example, he once surprised Abby at her office with enough pizza for her and her colleagues. After she angrily sent him away for disrupting her workplace, he brought the pizzas, an extravagant expense for him, to my apartment to breathlessly recount what had happened, eating almost all the slices himself. Later, Hải tried to enlist me in helping him recreate a scene involving cue cards from the film *Love Actually*.

In repeated conversations with me at cafés and restaurants over a period of several months, Hải attributed his behavior to the universal power of love. He gave me the same answers when I asked him, "Why do you love her?" and "How do you know you love her?": "I don't know. I just do." Yet he followed cultural scripts of chivalry, care, and gender that were mapped onto his fantasies of the West and the transformative properties of romance. Hải's refusal to accept Abby's rejections reflects masculine ideals of perseverance and assertiveness that in other contexts would be valued. (His conduct was not far removed from how Trâm wished Danh would act.) He went to any event that Abby might also attend and would try to talk with her all night in the hopes of recreating their initial spark. When I translated the concept of "stalking" as *săn* (hunting) to describe how Abby might interpret his actions as threatening, Hải mistook it as a compliment. He exaggerated Vietnamese gender roles that highlight masculine determination and feminine passivity to command Abby's attention because he assumed that Westerners are more romantically assertive.

Most critical to Hải's romantic self-making project, however, was his numerous expatriate friends' courtship advice: "Act natural" and "Be yourself." These suggestions focus on finding a soulmate to complement one's individuality instead of someone to fulfill social obligations that contributed to collective functioning. Hải hoped to reveal his adoration for Abby as an essential component of his self, assuming that what Abby wanted most was to be loved. ("Everyone wants to be loved," he reasoned.) However, it seemed more likely that Hải projected his own need for recognition onto her. He felt passive in his inability to control his emotions, but this passivity can also be understood as a strategy to establish his longings' intensity. This devotion was supposed to demonstrate his willingness to care for her, so he was puzzled when Abby (and Ngọc) did not reciprocate his feelings despite their authenticity and purity.

A paradox in the experience of unrequited love is that the love object exists so vividly in the person's experience of him or her but may not even know that the person exists. Abby occasionally texted Hải after their awkward encounters to apologize for not speaking more. They often chatted online late into the night, and Hải wondered why he was unable to reproduce in person the rapport he had with her online. The mixed signals and ambiguous rejections of his advances extended Hải's hopes for a relationship as well as anxieties about his worthiness as a suitor and, since he defined his self by his love for her, his entire being. Perhaps most troubling was that he sought out a particular form of recognition from Abby, but at times it seemed that she did not recognize his existence at all. Love had become an individual self-making project that was hindered by the lack of an object to validate his emotion work.

Increasingly the principal means of accessing romance's utopian promises, anxiety has become a defining feature of romance under late capitalism. Lovers transcend relationship problems and racial, gender, and class hierarchies through an intense fusion of selves that creates a state of liminality. Liminality is the means through which capitalist formations become ingrained in the phenomenology of (Western) romance because lovers depart from the mundane (e.g., romantic getaways) to affirm each other's selves (Illouz 1997). Indeed, Hải (and Trâm) crafted new versions of themselves by imagining or provoking ruptures in quotidian rules and responsibilities. However, their liminality stems from a more profound source of anxiety than everyday deviations: the reworking of the boundaries of the self. As Hải's obsession grew, the divide between his emotions' intensity and how much he actually knew about Abby became evident even to him. While he attributed this disparity to love's cosmic powers, I argue that it created a more fertile plane for the projection of his desires and produced a perceived immediacy in his experiences of her in his consciousness. His monadic intersubjectivity simultaneously conflated and co-constructed the love and the love object, echoing Berlant's observation that desire "visits you as an impact from the outside and yet, inducing an encounter with your affects, makes you feel as though it comes from within you" (2012, 6).

Falling in Like

As Hải told others the story of him and Abby, he revised his feelings so that he no longer fell head over heels in love. Instead, he realized he had only "fallen in like," which established a gradient of romantic attachment spread across varying degrees of emotional intensity and rational thought.[17] Moreover, if "true love" was a stable foundation for the type of relationship that Hải wanted but seemed further out of reach with every stilted interaction he had with Abby, then his feelings for her could not be "love." However, reframing his emotions as "falling in like" proved unsuccessful as an attempt to reason himself out of his own suffering. He spent hours in the pool to distract himself, but the disparity between his growing physical strength and his continued emotional vulnerability exacerbated his feelings of being held in Abby's sway.

While Hải considered his feelings for Abby a fundamental component of his psyche, love and the way he privileged his emotions as a matter of self-definition also express an emerging class identity. Romantic love became an extension of his self-making project. Although his inability to rationalize the self could be construed as a limit of đổi mới's affective impact, the very impetus to do so reflects a middle-class subject formation wherein selfhood is defined in emotive terms (Tran 2015). That is, the drive toward self-mastery frames emotions as threats to rationality, and self-control becomes increasingly valued as private feelings are taken as primary sources of self-knowledge and understanding. In our conversations about Abby, Hải often asked me what his emotions meant, eager to discuss their significance and decipher his own psyche. His friends, increasingly impatient with his sulking, advised him to ignore his feelings, which he interpreted as their not acknowledging him, his problems, and his goals in life. If the emotions stand in for the core of one's being, then to dismiss his feelings as irrational is to reject Hải himself. The discourse of romantic love articulates an ideal of individuated selves that should be accepted by others, a powerful draw for someone who often felt misunderstood and attacked by friends and family. However, by listening to him as a friend and an anthropologist, thus validating him as a person, was I also enabling toxic behavior? Despite my intention to not tell people what to do, I tried convincing him to stop pursuing Abby, to no avail.

Hải's cruelly optimistic[18] attachment to Abby and what she represented became a referendum on the self. That is, he needed not only her recognition as a romantic partner but also a validation of what he was doing (or not) in Ho Chi Minh City. His academic performance suffered, and any resolutions to refocus his studies usually fizzled out, since coursework reminded him that a career in finance was not what he wanted for himself. A relationship with Abby would give Hải a sense of purpose to focus his energies and replace the anomie of the seemingly random events and interactions that constituted his everyday life in Ho Chi Minh City.[19] Endowing Abby with a transformative power anchored broader anxieties about the self, but she, or rather his savior fantasy of her, formed an unstable foundation for a self-making project. Anthropological theories of emotion typically highlight the multiple ways that people draw on their emotions as a way to understand how people make sense of the world and of themselves (Levy 1984). One's own emotions can also be used to understand others, insofar as self-understanding entails thoughts, feelings, and behaviors made meaningful in relation to others. However, in Hải's experience, love operated independently of him. A defining feature of his self, it had somehow become alien to him. While the objectification of Hải's feelings as love gave him a social identity as an unpragmatic romantic, it also impeded other forms of self-knowledge, including the rational, reflexive understanding that eluded him.

Back in his hometown for summer break, Hải reached the nadir of his (lack of) experiences with Abby. Trying to push her out of his consciousness without the myriad distractions of Ho Chi Minh City, he did not feel anything, only numbness and emptiness, something he found difficult to put into words. When I asked him if he thought the English phrase *to feel dead inside* was an apt descriptor, he agreed and went on to quote a line from the poem "Yêu" (Love) by Xuân Diệu, a leading figure of the *Thơ Mới* movement: "*Yêu là chết ở trong lòng một ít.*" To love is to die inside a little. The next line, which Hải did not quote, is "*Vì mấy khi yêu mà chắc được yêu?*" For when you love, can you be sure you're loved? That modernist poetry published in 1938 resonates with Hải's very contemporary predicament attests to modernity's long precedent in Vietnam. However, that his feelings became his primary site of self-understanding, regardless of their usefulness, reflects the emotional self-reflexivity increasingly demanded by *đổi mới* selfhood. As Hải predicted, his broken heart only diminished with time. By the time he learned that Abby and an American she had been dating for a few months were expecting a child, he took the news in stride. Several months later, he developed long-standing flirtations with a few expatriates before becoming involved in a casual sexual relationship with a French woman. Despite being self-consciously careful to avoid developing a strong emotional attachment to her, he was unwilling to continue seeing her when she refused to be monogamous with him. When I asked him if he had started seeing anyone else, he said, "You know me. I still have feelings for her."

CONCLUSION

Hải once told me to interview people about who their perfect partner is, what makes them happy, and what they want in life because, according to him, Vietnamese people always think about love. That *thinking* is used synonymously with *worrying* in Vietnam suggests the prevalence of love anxiety. Trâm and Hải did not understand their own feelings. Often calling herself "crazy" during this period, Trâm was surprised by her emotional volatility, even though her reactions to her circumstances were far more measured than Hải's. While Trâm used romance to adapt to new circumstances, Hải sought outright transformation. If Trâm's case speaks to the convergence of anxiety and love, his suggests their co-emergence from the same underlying structures—social, political, and psychological. For him, love and anxiety were not just coexistent but also coterminous. In reevaluating the self according to the demands of emerging romantic discourses, Ho Chi Minh City's middle class can draw from a growing array of discourses of emotion, gender, and marriage. Doing so confronts them with alternative models of selfhood in the hybrid forms that romantic love takes in Vietnam. For many, holding up their current situations to such ideals is not only anxiety-inducing; their experience of romantic love is anxious itself.

For Ho Chi Minh City's emerging middle class, love is paradigmatic of the newfound freedoms and joys to be explored in the reform era (Nguyen 2007; Shohet 2017). However, reducing romantic love to a neoliberal self-making project ignores the role of other regimes of selfhood in the construction of modernist identities. Romance in Vietnam is a hybrid of various discourses of emotion, gender, and class, and the contradictions within this assemblage subsequently create anxieties about the self. Not simply the byproducts of romance, such anxieties are critical to the development, structure, and experience of romance itself. Indeed, they may compel people to adopt the hallmarks of neoliberal selfhood as much as, if not more than, the emotional intimacy that more typically characterizes romance.

However, love does not only belong to a subject. It is directed toward someone else with a particular set of properties. Love is in many respects "a giving over of a part of our being to another, or the self-estrangement of our being in its intimate entanglement with another" (Throop 2010a, 774). Unsurprisingly, neither Trâm nor Hải believed they could enact alternative selves on their own. This required another person, a love object, to become who they wanted to be. Given the foreign notions of romantic love they used to accommodate ideal versions of themselves, it is perhaps no coincidence that Westerners, real and imagined, figured in the goals of both. Neoliberal models of the emotions frame them as the ultimate source of self-knowledge. However, love anxiety does not just stem from people's changed relations to others or even their changed positions in contemporary Vietnamese society. Rather, it stems from a changed perception of their own selves that has been rendered unrecognizable to them by romantic love, a project of both self-making and self-alienation. Anxiety is both the author and remainder of romantic self-making projects.

When my initial fieldwork ended, Trâm was still married. Given her tendency to interpret emotions through a behavioral frame, I suspected that she justified her decision to stay married as one motivated by love: her apparent inability to initiate divorce proceedings must be evidence of love. This could be read as either the triumph of marital love over infidelity or, more cynically, anxiety over starting a new life. However, the next time I saw her, three years later, she and Danh were markedly different, "in love" even. She reported that they understood each other better because they now communicated their anger instead of keeping it to themselves. When I asked her if they were happy together, Trâm laughed. "I don't know."

7

How We Worry

I have never been more anxious than when I was writing the first draft of this concluding chapter, but the reason had little to do with the book. By the closing months of 2020, millions of people worldwide had died from COVID-19. Beyond the health and humanitarian devastations, virtually every aspect of our lives changed beneath our feet. Global industries and institutions abruptly ground to a halt, and anchors of everyday routines, such as work, school, and socializing, slipped into flashpoints of uncertainty. My home country of the United States, which accounted for a quarter of the cases of infection and had one of the highest death rates in the world, also had to contend with the social unrest and widespread protests over racialized police violence and the erosion of democratic norms. Breathless predictions that the social order will never be the same abounded, but the sheer variety and intensity of social changes compounding one another made it difficult to even begin processing the implications. Without a single, clear point of orientation, anxiety attacks from all directions. What Freud and Kierkegaard described as the internal structure of anxiety had become mimicked by the state of the world. People typically experience anxiety from within, but it sometimes seemed as if I existed inside anxiety itself.

As the global severity of the novel coronavirus became apparent in March 2020, researchers, politicians, journalists, and activists alike called for attention to the mental health effects of both the pandemic and the lockdown measures. Indeed, in the United States, mental health concerns would go on to become a political football in debates over public health measures aimed at containing or mitigating the spread of SARS-CoV-2. Many predicted that the pandemic would create a shadow epidemic of mental illness and that the mental health consequences of the pandemic will linger in communities longer than the physical health ones. The economic fallout of the pandemic exacerbated well-known risk factors for mental illness, including job and food insecurity, domestic violence, and social isolation. Vulnerable populations already contending with structural violence and racial and gender inequality are at even higher risk for mental health problems yet have the least access to resources for treatment (WHO 2014; Lund et al. 2018).

Meanwhile, despite sharing a common border and extensive bilateral trade with China, where the SARS-CoV-2 virus first emerged, Vietnam became one of the great success stories of the pandemic. When the first case of COVID-19 was recorded on January 23, 2020, several public health measures to curb infections were immediately—and successfully—implemented. Until the first coronavirus-related death was reported seven months later, Vietnam had been the largest country in the world with no such fatalities. It was also one of the few countries in the world to achieve economic growth in 2020.[1] Some American politicians and pundits, bemoaning the fact that the wealthiest country in the world could mount such an inadequate response to the pandemic, noted that "even Vietnam" outperformed the United States. Ho Chi Minh City residents returned to offices, restaurants, and each other's homes, albeit with some social distancing measures still in place. Many of my friends reached out to me, asking me if my family and I were safe, how we were coping with stay-at-home orders, and whether or not I would receive a federal stimulus check. They expressed pity (*tội nghiệp*) toward my fellow Americans. Notwithstanding the periodic flashes of research-related panic and insecurity, I confess that my interest in Ho Chi Minh City residents' *anxieties* was largely academic. At times, the landscape of my interlocutors' collective anxieties seemed as foreign to me as anything in my fieldsite. Until now.

A critical evaluation of a supposedly impending epidemic of anxiety, however, is required not in spite of its self-evident nature but rather because of it (Baxter et al. 2014). Claims of an epidemic or disaster often serve as pretext for state and humanitarian interventions (Redfield 2005; Seale-Feldman 2020). While intense anxiety may be a symptom of an underlying disorder, it is a problem only if the worrisome feelings are not justified or advantageous. Certainly, a once-in-a-century pandemic is as good an occasion as any for anxiety. For example, hypervigilance and increased attention to detail help people navigate once-familiar routines that have suddenly become potential vectors of a novel coronavirus. Most people demonstrate resilience in the face of natural and humanitarian disasters and political and social unrest, and such crises do not necessarily drive increases in mental illness (Argenti-Pillen 2003; Fassin and Rechtman 2009). Indeed, the very real suffering from a broad range of adversity that most people experience can be addressed without a diagnosis and costly treatment from medical specialists (Rose 2019).

Moreover, alarm over anxiety had already been growing before the pandemic's onset. As we contend with a profound insecurity about the future and a resulting sense of unease, anxiety has become perhaps the dominant affective key through which we experience and interpret our personal lives and our collective movements. The global rise of the psy-disciplines and biomedical diagnoses and treatments for anxiety disorders have created new conceptual tools to rethink people's approach to overthinking, neurasthenia, and *nervios*, among other conditions. Thus, the intense focus on anxiety in recent years should be read as part of a

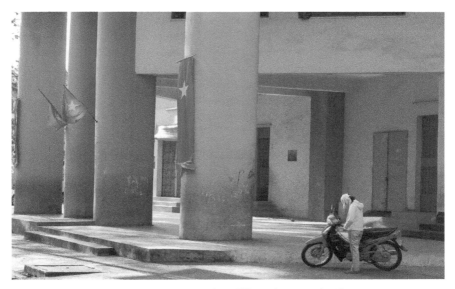

FIGURE 6. A motorist in District 5 protects herself from the sun and pollution.

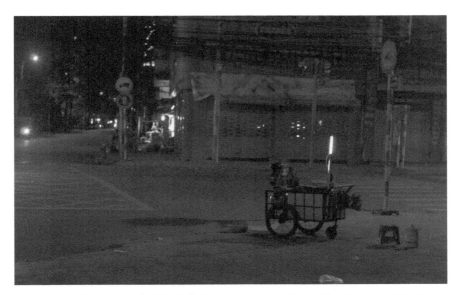

FIGURE 7. A fluorescent tube light bulb draws attention to a late-night air pump in District 3.

broader psychologization of everyday life. Of course, people have often spent much of their day discussing their feelings. However, the present moment is marked by a sheer density of emotion in public discourse in which situations, events, and institutions are assessed mainly in terms of their affective impacts (Lerner and Rivkin-Fish 2021). Now taken as the crux of authenticity, the emotions have become sites of moral reckoning and experiments with personhood (Béhague and MacLeish 2020). However, the affective mode of these self-making projects is an anxious one. No wonder the end result is so often prone to worry. Anxiety may not be just one particular manifestation of the emotionalization of public life but rather a consequence of it. Do we find ourselves in a particularly uncertain era, or have we found in anxiety a salient trope to make sense of it? Or, perhaps most troubling, is the vantage point from which we take in uncertainty part of the problem?

AN AGENDA FOR FUTURE RESEARCH

If an age of global anxiety is upon us (Zhang 2020), the work of tracing its reach calls for a cross-cultural framework for anxiety that attributes as much significance to the details of its context as to the intricacies of its experience. Thus, to conclude this book, I propose a collaborative agenda for future research and practice on anxiety and associated disorders that links the personal and the political. Market reforms and the resulting inner turn have rendered insecurities increasingly reflexive and challenge our understandings of the self as the subject of politics (Burgess 2017). Working against the reductionist argument that anxiety is the unavoidable product of economic reforms captures rather than reproduces the neoliberal logic that emotions are apolitical. By highlighting how economic transformations and the psychic experience of anxiety mutually reinforce each other, a perspective from critical phenomenology bridges the material and immaterial, the discursive and the bodily, and the clinical and the political. Given that subjectivity is a matter of engagement with and attunement to the world, the self does not simply perceive external dangers and then react to them with anxiety. Unlike the presumably autonomous and sovereign self that defines neoliberal subjectivity, this understanding of selfhood is always on the cusp of becoming undone, and risk is inseparable from who and what we are. Below, I outline some overlapping threads that frame the mutual constitution and reconstitution of the social and the psychic in a way that places anxiety at the center of the analysis of political transformations. These broad themes—the sources, discourse, experience, and politics of anxiety— are far from exhaustive or complete. Rather, I intend this to be a starting point of a necessary and long-overdue conversation.

The Sources of Anxiety

The starting point for our ethnographic framework for anxiety is identifying the primary sources of people's worries. After all, they are already common topics of discussion. "Troubles talk" and similar conversational genres feature heavily in everyday sociality as people seek out instrumental, social, and emotional support (Garro 2003; Wilce 2003; Pritzker 2020). Identifying people's worries not only becomes a means of becoming acquainted and further engaging with people but also sheds insight into their concerns and perceived vulnerabilities.

While anthropologists have often noted their interlocutors' anxieties, the analytic focus tends to be on the causes of anxiety as a means to investigate broader social changes. What distinguishes ethnographic research specifically on anxiety from research that takes people's anxieties into account is attention to how people understand and grapple with anxiety and how anxiety shapes social action. Relying on explicit discussions and self-reports about people's worries admittedly highlights those anxieties that are readily articulated in public forms and settings. Yet silence can be deployed strategically, and much can be gleaned from what is unsaid and kept private in these conversations (Searles 2000). Recognizing the local cues of troubles talk requires that researchers identify and adopt the modes of moral personhood and care that form the existential ground of anxiety (Csordas et al. 2010).

Documenting a community's collective fearscapes and outlining their general pattern reveals the uncertain futures that people orient toward. How people react to new insecurities reflects what matters most to them and reveals long-standing but previously concealed social tensions. Indeed, these anxieties may become flashpoints in debates about the proper social order. For example, Ho Chi Minh City's fearscape of family and financial pressures is oftentimes so mundane to its residents that they seem too bored to discuss any of these fears in depth. Rather, they are more keen to marvel at the general differences between the anxieties of the past and those that dominate the present. When Ho Chi Minh City residents say that they worry more than ever before, perhaps what they mean is that they have more things to worry about. Here, not only the sources of anxiety but their general pattern is important to note. In post-reform Vietnam, everyday life has diversified. People must keep track of and navigate new types of people, occupations, and material goods that have come into the city. In combination, these distinct worries, even if the stakes are less dire than they were before economic reforms, exacerbate each other. Thus, the structure and rhythm of everyday life in the reform era has led to pervasive anxiety and alienation. That concerns about emerging trends and technologies are articulated through a prism of modernity and progress indicates that the sources of anxiety become meaningful in relation to other discourses.

The Discourse of Anxiety

It is not just the content of people's worries that shifts during an emerging age of anxiety. How they make sense of and talk about anxiety also reflects the social changes that spark novel forms of anxiety. Simply put, new causes of concern call for new ways of understanding them. Dominant frameworks for anxiety tend to ignore how and what people think about their worries. For example, epidemiological studies of anxiety and anxiety disorders usually attempt to determine the relative quantity of anxiety across communities or historical periods (Baxter et al. 2013, 2014). The degree to which these measures are cross-culturally valid is limited by the biases of the researchers themselves. Unsurprisingly, these measures of anxiety reflect Western folk theories of the emotions that frame them primarily in biological and, hence, universally applicable terms (Lutz 1988). These determinations are possible only when the conceptualizations of anxiety by those who suffer from it are disregarded, standardized, and generalized across cultural and historical contexts.

Because anxiety can be such a confounding and vague experience, people often resort to a variety of discourses to make sense of it. In their attempts to do so, people also articulate their vision of the social order. As such, this process always operates in the context of power dynamics that elevate some experiences—and some people—over others. Here, I discuss two common discourses of anxiety in Vietnam that are widespread globally: modernity and medicalization. Conversations about anxiety in many parts of the world have long drawn on discourses of modernity and progress (Tone 2008; Tran 2016). Whether as a result of *đổi mới* policies, the electrical age, or social media, they construct anxiety as a recent phenomenon, suggesting that an anxious person is also a modern one. Understanding how other ages of anxiety are tied to notions of progress and of living too fast sheds light on the hidden logics that animate the moral panics that so often surround anxiety.

It is tempting to dismiss Vietnam's age of anxiety as outright impossible, given the counterintuitive premise that as people's economic fortunes improve, so have the range and magnitude of their anxieties. After all, why would people worry more during a period of economic and technological progress? Who has the right to complain about being anxious? Many of the people who told me some version of the "age of anxiety" story were younger members of Ho Chi Minh City's rising middle class, which suggests that it may be a self-congratulatory narrative that validates the packed schedules of social and economic elites (such as academics!), as proof of how important they are and how taxing their work is. Rising rates of anxiety disorders in Vietnam are folded into a wider narrative of the discovery of a more authentic way of living from the West.

Notions of progress also animate another discourse of anxiety that has become globally popular: its medicalization. The biomedical doctrine that everyday suffering and emotional distress can be understood as a health problem and treated as such has become perhaps the dominant framework for mental health and illness in the world. Despite its ubiquity and hegemony, however, biomedical psychiatry has not entirely replaced indigenous ways of coping with extreme anxiety. Rather, biomedical encounters with local systems of meaning produce hybridized forms of diagnosing and treating psychic distress. By documenting how people interpret biomedical theories of mental illness in relation to their existing understandings, researchers can push back against narratives of the inevitability of modern medicine replacing "traditional" healing practices. Thus, cross-cultural research is needed to investigate the broad range of anxiety disorders that do not conform to the *DSM*'s diagnostic criteria and to better understand the relation between anxiety disorders and normative levels and types of anxiety (Clark 1987; Fabrega 1990). Ethnographic studies of the cultural specificities of disordered anxiety can inform more general research on mental illness by triangulating with epidemio-logical and clinical research (Lopez and Guarnaccia 2000). How is abnormal anxi-ety determined in different societies? Is intense anxiety a universal form of mental illness? Is it even usefully understood as pathology?

The emergence of an anxiety-specific genre of troubles talk reflects the ongoing effort to normalize struggles with mental health. Ho Chi Minh City's psy-experts seek to boost mental health literacy by disseminating psychotherapeutic concepts and techniques in online and offline fora. Many middle-class Vietnamese youth have taken keen interest in psychology as a field of study and increasingly frame mental health and emotional self-knowledge as key to living the good life. For example, when I asked a Ho Chi Minh City–based college student if she considered herself an adult yet, she said no, because she still relied on her parents to financially sup-port her, but that she was more of an adult than her "alcoholic" parents who never reflected on, let alone understood, their own feelings. For her and many of her peers in Vietnam and the West (Silva 2012), mental health has become a marker of matu-rity, echoing trends among American youth. However, attempts to destigmatize mental illness by portraying it as an illness like any other have thus far not absolved individual sufferers of responsibility and blame (Rose 2019). Framing mental ill-ness as a generic illness reinforces the notion that emotional distress is located within the brain and should be treated individually with approaches such as medi-cation or psychotherapy, instead of focusing on structural measures. This reflects the professionalization of care as medical experts assume greater authority over patients and their family caregivers. Moreover, current efforts to normalize mental illness focus on a narrow range of disorders. For example, in recent years, men-tal health awareness campaigns attempt to destigmatize anxiety and mood disor-ders far more than schizoaffective disorders. The subtext is clear: it is easier to get anxious and depressed individuals back to maximum productivity through treat-ments that do not require significant adjustments to their surroundings.

The Experience of Anxiety

What the sources, concepts, and discourses of anxiety share in common is that they play out perhaps most profoundly at the level of the self. Discourse not only reveals the ways in which anxiety is felt, but also constructs its very presence, and attend-ing to the body uncovers what is left unsaid. Although biomedical psychiatry tends to dismiss physical complaints as secondary to a psychiatric diagnosis, headaches, insomnia, or exhaustion, among others, should not be ignored because somatic idioms of distress express both personal distress and political conflict. For example, when open complaints lead to social conflict, anxiety is often somatized due to dif-ficult relationships and persistent experiences of suffering and pain (Hinton and Hinton 2002). The body mediates the social dynamics that often lead to chronic mental illness, and chronic somatization links the local meanings of emotional dis-tress to the physiology of illness (Good and Kleinman 2019; Csordas 1993).

In many parts of the world, the increasing reliance on the psy-disciplines to assuage our worried minds shifts not just how people cope with anxiety but also how they manage their emotions and understandings of themselves. The growth of the psychotherapeutic and wellness industries in neoliberalizing contexts often commodifies emotional intimacy and pathologizes precarity (Illouz 2008; Matza 2018). For example, discourses that promote self-sufficiency also cultivate a highly emotive self that explores its own inner anxieties as a matter of self-discovery. In their therapeutic encounters, Ho Chi Minh City residents are encouraged to attend to and label their private feelings in order to articulate them to others. In doing so, they learn that the emotions are an ever-present undercurrent of their stream of consciousness and social experiences. Because of the vulnerability inherent to being open to any and all emotions, however, enacting these forms of selfhood may court anxiety more than other affective experiences. Increasingly popular ideas about emotion, morality, and the good life are made possible by the cultivation of a self that is directed inward. Their increasing presence in everyday life may not just reflect a growing demand for relief from anxiety. Indeed, it may be part of the problem.

Collective institutions once used to define the self have become profoundly transformed. Instead, selfhood is increasingly reinvented on an individual basis as people try new ways of conceptualizing and coping with chronic anxiety. Today, the renegotiation of people's worries is most clearly articulated within therapeutic contexts, such as psychiatric clinics, pharmacies, and counseling centers. However, conflicting ways of drawing the boundary between normative and pathological anxiety are no less vociferous in the more mundane settings of work and leisure throughout the city. When people try to determine how-much-is-too-much, Ho Chi Minh City residents are not just engaged in an effort to alter their anxieties. Unwittingly or not, they effectively transform their own selves. Anxiety stems from how people have adapted to and interface with a rapidly changing socioeconomic environment that has fundamentally altered previous means of grappling with life's difficulties. Not only is the self the primary terrain on which anxiety plays out, it has become the source of its own torment. Could relying on the emotions—or even the concept of emotion itself—to construct their identities create new models of identity? How might the global call for mental health awareness contribute to a new form of identity politics, one that is less rooted in the neurodiversity movement (Singer 1999; Silberman 2015) than in a form of psy-diversity?

The Politics of Anxiety

Anxiety registers not just at a bodily level but at a political one as well, making its politics inseparable from its meaning and experiential force (Burgess 2017). The fact that anxiety is usually regarded as a byproduct of political economy is, in and of itself, indicative of a political order that is disguised as something decidedly apolitical. Recognizing that it is "only human" to be anxious in the precarious

situations in which so many of us find ourselves in the twenty-first century naturalizes emerging subjectivities. Indeed, "authenticity" under neoliberalism may, in
fact, be cover for "neoliberal authoritarianism" (Neocleous 2017). Taking anxiety
seriously as a productive form of politics illuminates how it shapes us as political
subjects (Eklundh, Guittet, and Zevnik 2017). Instead of trying to prevent, limit, or
overcome anxiety, we should attempt to understand its role in the political order.

The dual rise of anxiety and economic prosperity in Vietnam challenges persistent assumptions about the assumed relation between progress and a better life, as
well as the neoliberal fantasy of self-fulfilled subjects. The painful effects of development schemes are often justified with assurances that a wealthy population will
be a healthy and happy one, but the age of anxiety questions long-held assumptions about anxiety and its relation to progress and the good life, selfhood and suffering, and mood and morality. Having come to define the subjective experience
of global and national processes, anxiety is not an aberration on the road to progress or its unfortunate byproduct. Rather, as it gets taken up in new self-making
projects, anxiety is itself implicated in Vietnam's socioeconomic transformation.
Examining how various forms of worry are being recoded reveals how anxiety is
embedded in neoliberal forms of modernity as part of a dialectical relationship
between the self and the larger political economy.

Anxiety is a political practice because it informs, embodies, and ultimately
enables a logic of security (Rossi 2017).[2] Oriented toward the unknown, anxiety
emerges from anticipations about the future. It is the product of what has yet to
happen, of the worst to come, rather than something that is "over and done with."
In a society organized around risk, this constant sense of unease is not an objective fact but rather is nurtured (Beck 1992). At the heart of self-making projects
that prepare for future threats is cultivating vigilance to guard against precarity
and, crucially, the coping mechanisms to deal with it. People come to expect that
threats may happen and learn to cope with them on an individual basis through,
for example, psychotherapeutically informed practices. Indeed, they may even
be required to be collectively anxious yet individually resilient but not politically
mobilized (Neocleous 2017; Yang 2015). The result is a deeply anxious subjectivity that is endlessly constructed through the prospect that things could always
get worse.

. . .

Vietnam's age of anxiety is the result of both new forms of insecurity and new
ways of responding to them. To meet the demands of the reform economy, Ho
Chi Minh City's middle class increasingly turn to the psy-disciplines as a guide
through the widening possibilities for their lives. In particular, the emotions have
come to stand for the contradictions of modern selfhood. Rising rates of anxiety
disorders reflect burgeoning expectations of the good life as well as long-standing
concerns about gendered morality. In learning to manage their anxieties, Ho Chi

Minh City residents expand their emotional repertoire as a matter of self-discovery instead of only attending to the feelings of others because they depend on them for basic survival. However, as a result, people are caught between overlapping frames of emotion, sentiment, and selfhood and must reconcile competing models of worry: a form of care or an obstacle to self-realization and fulfillment. For many Ho Chi Minh City residents, coping with the pressures, deadlines, and conflicts of the reform era may lead to different but no less profound anxieties of the self. Indeed, the foundations of selfhood—the very means through which people respond to anxiety—have been called into question, perhaps helpfully for some, by the tools used to cope with this new world of uncertainty. At a time when people across the globe increasingly turn to the pharmaceutical and wellness industries to soothe their troubled minds, it is worth considering whether the social and political dynamics that make them an appealing salve to begin with may be partly to blame.

In Vietnam and beyond, anxiety has become a key signifier of neoliberal subjectivities and one of the most popular guides through our present precarity. The rise of anxiety in public life is evidence of both increasingly common forms of uncertainty and vulnerability and the complexity of the global and human interconnectedness of the current moment. The way we respond to the new age of anxiety should reflect that, but thus far it does not. Insofar as its discourses shape how we understand and resolve the emotional concerns of ourselves and those around us, the psy-disciplines have become insinuated with "the very experience of living" (Rose 2019, 3). If anxiety is indeed both a social practice and a social condition, this has different implications for what should be done to address the impending age of global anxiety. From this perspective, anxiety is not simply something to be managed and controlled, and it cannot be treated away with pharmaceutical interventions or tamped down with therapeutic techniques and principles. The biomedical impulse to eliminate anxiety from our lives may cause more harm than good if we do not ask what function anxiety performs. Cross-cultural research can reveal alternative perspectives on how anxiety operates in disparate social contexts. This is not to deny the very real benefits and even pleasures that many find in psychiatry. Indeed, many Ho Chi Minh City residents found the process of self-discovery to be liberating from toxic and dysfunctional relationships. However, if people use therapeutic ideals and techniques to extricate themselves from difficult affective entanglements, we should also ask what they free them to.

Mental health treatments are undoubtedly needed around the world, and training more mental health workers to meet the demands of ever more diverse communities is critical. Public mental health measures that are derived from the psy-disciplines will likely have minimal effect if the underlying social determinants of mental health and illness are ignored (Rose et al. 2020). Addressing rising rates of anxiety disorders and mental health inequities more broadly requires attention to the political and economic factors that drive ill health through a structurally informed course of action. Even the World Health Organization (WHO), which has long promoted global mental health through Western standards of care, recently critiqued an overreliance on biomedical treatments and endorsed a structural approach to reforming mental health treatment around the world (WHO 2021). A fundamental rethinking of mental health care is under way, and anthropologists are well positioned to investigate, assess, and design programs that link individual healing and structural transformation through community mental health.

Because strong social ties and forms of relatedness are better predictors of mental health than individual satisfaction (Turner, Frankel, and Levin 1983), public health measures should enhance social support, solidarity, and equity (Quinn, Bromage, and Rowe 2020) as well as resources that enhance the realization of one's own capabilities (Hopper 2007). Thus, therapeutic interventions for individuals should be positioned as part of an overall strategy toward systemic change. Such structural transformations may reduce the currently overwhelming need for mental health care services (Hodgetts and Stolte 2017). Emphasizing collective forms of belonging and citizenship counterbalances therapeutic governance and its emphasis on individuated treatments by prioritizing people's participation in society over managing their own treatment and personal stability (Myers, Lester, and Hopper 2016). However, social solidarity is no simple antidote to the individuating effects of neoliberal policies. No doubt a reaction to the isolation and separation that many experienced during COVID-19 lockdowns, the recent romanticization of collectivism and calls for community often veer into exoticization and condescension. They also ignore how ideals such as self-care or emotional intelligence can be used to nurture familial and community networks (Pritzker and Duncan 2019). Moreover, many Ho Chi Minh City residents sought treatment and support from the psy-disciplines because of the burdens of caring for others. The relational forms of selfhood and care that are so often idealized by Vietnamese themselves depend on inequalities as some shoulder the expectations for sacrifice more than others (Shohet 2021).

Anxiety need not only limit our politics. Conceptualizing anxiety as a social practice that creates relationships based on care allows us to reimagine the relationship between anxiety and politics. By disrupting political subjectivities, anxiety can alter the reach of the state. What if anxiety as a tool of governance were oriented not toward an individual ethics of autonomy and sovereignty, but rather toward a relational ethics of care (Stevenson 2014)? How can anxiety be mobilized to shift political structures to treat people as relational beings in addition to autonomous individuals? Framing anxiety as a moral sentiment of care and concern invites an ethical attunement to the Other. This approach, both ethical and political, builds alternative possibilities for being together (Zigon 2021). As global pandemics and political divisions have sparked and renewed our fears of each other, we need to find ways to foreground our relationships and what we are to each other. Instead of turning inward to cope with our worries, pursuing meaningful social relationships and collective action instead not only soothes our troubled minds but also works against the capitalist logic of self-determination that has frayed community bonds and made us feel so vulnerable in the first place. Uncertainty is connected to an openness to the future, and anxiety is evidence of the possibilities, dangers, and freedoms in how we constitute and reconstitute ourselves in response to what comes next.

1. HOW TO WORRY

1. This form of happiness refers to a sense of positive happenstance, similar to the original meaning of the word *happy* in English.

2. Different types of anxiety disorders themselves have proliferated in the *DSM*, due to the shift toward behaviors as the basis of diagnostic categories as well as the increased use of selective serotonin reuptake inhibitors (SSRIs), formerly used primarily as an antidepressant, to treat a wider variety of maladies, extending pharmaceutical companies' patents in the process (Horwitz 2010).

3. To be sure, the notion that anxieties take on a life of their own when they can no longer be managed by one's own conscious effort reflects a Western model of personhood that locates its core in self-control and its ability to reason. To construct the formation of anxiety as a biographical subject is one means of imposing order on its chaos and unruliness. Yet the model of the person as a rational, bounded entity holds an ambivalent position in this book. To point out its Western biases, I rely on data on how people in Vietnam claim it as their own; the more I deconstruct the liberal subject, the harder it seems to leave behind.

4. For exceptions, see Lloyd and Moreau (2011) and Middleton (2013).

5. A common critique of the Party entails comparisons to South Korea and Singapore. In 1975, Vietnam was more well developed than either of those countries, yet their economic indicators now far surpass those of Vietnam. It should be noted, however, that South Korea's economic success was due, in large part, to US investment in the economy during the 1980s that was promised in return for South Korea's military support during the Second Indochina War.

6. According to Bourke (2005), the "fearscapes" of preindustrial societies tend to be dominated by specific dangers to life and limb. As the material gains and comforts of modernity reduce the threat of sudden death, generalized anxieties about a loss of social and economic status suffuse postindustrial fearscapes.

7. Although I distinguish between the emotions as a set of discrete feeling states (e.g., happiness and anger) and affect as a felt bodily intensity, I focus on their overlap. Characterizing affect as concerned with inchoate feelings, and emotion as concerned with expression and meaning, reifies Cartesian dichotomies of mind and body or reason and passion. Moreover, since affect and emotion share an ethnopsychological context, the frequent slippages between them can make such distinctions difficult.

8. Later generations of psychodynamically oriented theorists would focus on how anxiety emerges from people's attempts to relate themselves to others (Klein 1948; Lacan 2016).

9. See Ewing (1990) for a discussion of selfhood and notions of wholeness.

10. Ho Chi Minh City has a reputation for being open to change and foreign influence, and the trends described here may be more similar to other large cities in Southeast Asia (Jones 2004) than to the rest of Vietnam.

11. The availability of choices opens the possibilities of fulfilling our desires, but psychological research indicates that excessive amounts of options in terms of snacks, entertainments, career paths, and romantic partners can overwhelm us into depression and anxiety. In *The Paradox of Choice*, Schwartz argues against the idea that increasing choice will create more freedom and that freedom should be equated with happiness.

12. That Ngọc Bình is based in Hanoi suggests that the turn toward the psy-disciplines has spread from Ho Chi Minh City to other urban centers in Vietnam. Many Ho Chi Minh City–based psychotherapists believe themselves to be at the vanguard of their field in the country.

13. Ngọc Bình [@ngocbinhtamly], "Bạn căng thẳng sau một tuần? DÀNH CHO BẠN!," *TikTok*, March 21, 2021, https://www.tiktok.com/@ngocbinhtamly/video/6941351 678897622273?is_from_webapp = 1&sender_device = pc&web_id = 7128865888747324974.

14. Ngọc Bình [@ngocbinhtamly], "Mình chỉ muốn nói là trên TikTok còn rất nhiều người sẵn sàng cho b những lời khuyên bổ ích," *TikTok*, June 11, 2021, https://www.tiktok .com/@ngocbinhtamly/video/6972388573060320514?is_from_webapp = 1&sender_device = pc&web_id = 7128865888747324974.

15. Despite the growing specialization and sophistication in how people describe psychiatric conditions, many still confuse the terms for depression and autism. What links these diagnoses together is an imagined withdrawal from sociality that is most pathologized.

16. The psychologist Abraham Maslow (1943) posited that humans have a universal hierarchy of needs, and that individuals are motivated to secure their physiological and safety needs, such as food and shelter, before addressing their psychological and self-fulfillment needs, such as feelings of love and fame. According to him, people afraid of starving to death are too busy to worry about higher-order concerns about self-actualization. From this perspective, the stress of choosing a career path that not only meets one's physiological needs with a steady income, but also meets one's self-actualization goals with professional fulfillment, is a testament to historical and economic progress. While Maslow's theory broadly makes sense, its rigid progression of needs reflects middle-class Western values of individualism. For example, in the hierarchy of needs, physical security comes before belonging to a social group. However, belonging to a social group may be a requirement in order to achieve security. Moreover, the lack of cultural variability reflects a universalist emphasis on individual psychology and a glossing-over of social structure.

2. MORAL SENTIMENTS

1. Expressions of constant thinking that communicate emotional distress have led some anthropologists to argue that the Vietnamese do not distinguish between cognition and emotion (Cadiere 1957; Rydstrøm 2003a; Gammeltoft 1999). However, Vietnamese strongly differentiate between the passions and rationality, albeit in ways that do not overlap in the exact same ways as Western dualisms. Descriptions of psychic states may combine worry with other states to produce an effect that decreases the distance between cognitive and affective activity, but they remain distinct. For example, *buồn lo* (sad and worried) features worry as a cognitive anchor, and *lo nghĩ* (worried thinking) features it as an affective descriptor. It is perhaps this "imprecise" way of expressing psychic activity that led Cadiere to conclude that Vietnamese cannot distinguish thought and emotion.

2. The words for "real" or "realistic" and "practical" or "pragmatic" are the same in Vietnamese: *thực tế*.

3. Bayly (2020) similarly notes that Hanoians characterize Westerners as rational and rule-bound and Vietnamese as emotional and committed to other people.

4. These observations of northerners and southerners feed into their stereotypes of each other. Northerners consider southerners to have too much *tình cảm* and therefore to be not as diligent and frugal as northerners fancy themselves. Meanwhile, southerners stereotype northerners' relative lack of *tình cảm* as reason for their untrustworthiness and inability to take the risks in building the necessary long-term relationships needed to compete in the market economy.

5. The disproportionate burden of worries that women bear in Vietnamese society stems from several sources, including a Confucian legacy of patriarchal authority, the moral ambivalence about petty commercial trading that is traditionally seen as an extension of women's domestic prowess (Pettus 2003; Leshkowich 2014a; Leshkowich and Endres 2018), high rates of domestic violence (Horton and Rydstrøm 2011), and stricter ethical standards for women (Rydstrøm 2003a; Gammeltoft 1999), among others.

6. This parallels Shohet's observation that sacrifice (*hy sinh*) is discursively divided into a state-sanctioned rhetoric of masculinist patriotism and an unofficial version of feminine virtues regarding familial care (2021).

7. This paragon is reflected in Nguyễn Du's nineteenth-century epic poem "The Tale of Kiều" (*Truyện Kiều*), perhaps Vietnam's most famous literary classic. The poem recounts the trials of a woman who sacrifices herself as a courtesan for her family and symbolizes the endurance and resilience of the Vietnamese (Tan 2016).

8. Most Vietnamese youth live with their parents until they get married. However, in recent years, young members of Ho Chi Minh City's rising middle class have increasingly sought out independent living arrangements.

3. RICH SENTIMENTS

1. Schwenkel (2012) notes that the word *emotion* appears in English in Vietnamese advertisements for Vespa motorbikes.

2. Harms (2009) examines sidewalk cafés' status in the city's public and increasingly privatized spaces.

3. This is not to deny the importance of emotion's newfound associations with consumerism. Self-fashioning as modern Vietnamese through consumption is encouraged within state-determined parameters, marking a shift from the immediate postwar era (1975–86), when consumerism was antithetical to socialist morality. Currently, commercial activity has become further dissociated from the state and legitimates state authority by depoliticizing consumption and the self-work involved therein. The state is heavily invested in the production of subjectivities through encouraging citizens to remake themselves in ways that promote state/market ideals (Leshkowich 2012; Vann 2012).

4. Greenhalgh and Winckler (2005) and Yan (2011) observe similar patterns in Chinese cities.

5. Throughout East and Southeast Asia, neoliberalism is associated with market economies, consumerism, and privatization as well as entry into free trade organizations like the World Trade Organization (Rofel 2007; Nonini 2008; Rudnyckyj 2011).

6. See Ots (1990).

7. For example, most of my interlocutors assumed that *thất tình* referred to "lovesickness," as *thất* refers to the number seven in Sino-Vietnamese and to "loss" in Vietnamese. Those who are aware of the seven emotions typically can only recall three or four items.

8. Spoken in English.

9. Space does not permit discussion of what English terms used to discuss emotion index in Vietnamese, but it should be noted that many of my respondents who spoke at length about *cảm xúc* are at least moderately proficient in English, a reflection of their mostly middle-class background.

10. Yan (2010) describes a similar shift from responsibilities to rights in China.

11. Tang (2000) and Yan (2011) note that Chinese discourses of everyday life have expanded to legitimize self-expression.

12. Although a prolonged period of bereavement before remarrying occurs in Vietnam, it is more expected of widows than of widowers and is idealized more often than actually practiced, since this Confucian valorization of spousal loyalty is predicated on a social order that no longer exists.

4. THE MEDICALIZATION OF WORRY

1. Ho Chi Minh City's public hospitals receive many patients from rural areas who travel hours or even days because they believe that urban hospitals offer more sophisticated treatments.

2. While many of the psychiatrists I knew in Ho Chi Minh City were themselves dubious of the study's methods and findings, they still acknowledged that large swaths of the country likely qualify for a psychiatric diagnosis.

3. The most prevalent psychiatric diagnoses in Vietnam are alcohol abuse (5.3%), depressive disorders (2.8%), and anxiety disorders (2.6%) (Ministry of Health 2002).

4. Some patients refer to neurasthenia as *suy nghĩ thần kinh* (nervous thinking) or *suy yếu thần kinh* (nervous weakness).

5. Panic among Cambodian refugees likewise entails neck pain (Hinton et al. 2006).

6. Twenty-five years after Kleinman's study at Hunan Medical University, Dere et al. (2013) found that doctors and patients there no longer used the diagnosis.

7. The sample consisted of thirty-four women and eleven men who were over eighteen years old and had received a diagnosis of GAD and/or MDD from their doctor. Here, I focus on anxiety-related dimensions of neurasthenia as patients emphasized symptoms related to worry over depression. However, there is considerable overlap because Vietnamese patients often blend anxiety and depressive disorders (Wagner et al. 2006).

8. This is partly due to how brief appointments are, as psychiatrists typically spend five to ten minutes with each patient due to high demand. Developing a relationship of trust between doctors and patients is also hindered by a general lack of privacy in the crowded wards and examination rooms. Patients at the outpatient psychiatric clinics at Army Hospital 175 and Nguyễn Trí Phương Hospital in Ho Chi Minh City do not have to compete as much for time and space as their counterparts at the Ho Chi Minh City Psychiatric Hospital. However, their doctor visits are comparable. According to patients, the primary benefit of these clinics over the psychiatric hospital is a shorter waiting time, not the standard of care.

9. Hoa also noted busying herself with domestic responsibilities when she was stressed. According to her, this is a more common strategy for rural women.

10. Contributing to psychiatry's poor reputation is that doctors are assigned their specialization according to their performance in medical school. Low-ranked students are directed toward psychiatry.

5. THE PSYCHOLOGIZATION OF WORRY

1. See Craciun (2018) for a sociological analysis of CBT.

2. Zhang (2018) notes a similar trend in China.

3. Therapists at other centers also had several children brought for treatment by their parents, only to find that the main culprit of the behavioral issue was the parents themselves. For example, Tuấn treated a boy who had been expelled from several schools for fighting. The cause of the fighting was not the boy's violent tendencies or anger issues. Rather, he was encouraged by his father, a member of the Communist Party, to always fight back against his enemies, the same way the Vietnamese resisted French and American forces.

4. Therapies that emphasize practical problem solving are generally more appealing to many Asian populations than psychodynamic treatments that focus on intrapsychic conflict (Hwang et al. 2006).

5. Indeed, this preference for concrete action is more widespread in Ho Chi Minh City than in other parts of Vietnam. During a break between panels at a mental health conference in Hanoi, Nguyên complained to me that the program reflected a distinctly Hanoian contemplativeness by focusing more on abstract theory than on specific practices.

6. Unsurprisingly, many of the pioneers of person-centered ethnographic interviewing have extensive clinical and ethnographic experience (Levy and Hollan 1988; Hollan 2001).

6. LOVE, ANXIETY

1. The woman relayed this story to me. I have never met Thịnh.

2. For example, in 2008, when I told people that I lived by myself, they usually asked me if I was sad/bored (*buồn*). As of this writing, however, young people increasingly choose to live by themselves if they can afford to live without roommates or apart from their families.

3. That motorbikes facilitate the culmination of this pair of vignettes is no accident. Motorbikes are part and parcel with many of the trends shaping the romantic dilemmas of Vietnam's growing middle class (Truitt 2008). The spatial and class mobility made possible by motorbikes poses new challenges for Thịnh and Trâm. Their respective trips to and from Ho Chi Minh City began as missions to escape or resolve worrisome situations yet ironically created more anxiety. In addition to motorbikes, underlying both of these stories (and the stories of many others) are profound uncertainties that undermine people's senses of self yet also extend and redefine their limits.

4. Shohet (2017) examines a case in which filial piety demands romantic love in central Vietnam.

5. Quinn (1987) draws on person-centered interviews to develop cultural models of marriage.

6. Trâm and Hải granted permission for research to examine their personal history and information.

7. This section's subheading is taken from Goode (1959).

8. Love has often been theorized as applicable to elites who have the requisite time to cultivate an aesthetic appreciation of subjective states (Stone 1977). That many of the trends described here are most germane to Ho Chi Minh City residents participating in an urban, consumerist lifestyle accords with this argument, but improved economic conditions are not sufficient to explain the particular forms that romantic love has taken.

9. Lee (2007) analyzes the role of romantic love in producing "modern" Chinese identities.

10. Spoken in English.

11. Indeed, *tình thương* means both "pity" and "affection" in Vietnamese.

12. Discourses of gender emphasize the restlessness of men's tastes (culinary and sexual) as a matter of instinct (Phinney 2008b; Rydstrøm 2003).

13. Modernization was seen as eroding the Vietnamese traditional family by causing both men and women to stray from their moral grounding and possibly destroy their families in the process (McGrath 2008).

14. Trâm seemed aware of this tension and was careful to avoid seeming materialistic. For women in market societies, love is both "a strategic choice and a refuge from market strategies" (Farrer 2002, 192; cf. Collier 1997).

15. Incidentally, he and Thiện are cousins.

16. I never met Abby. Hải conveyed these interactions to me.

17. Even minor instances of romantic interest or infatuation can be labeled love in Vietnamese.

18. See Berlant (2012).

19. Indeed, his fixation on a Westerner implies a greater rupture from everyday life than one on a Vietnamese woman would.

7. HOW WE WORRY

1. After several months-long stretches of "zero COVID," however, the arrival of the Delta variant in April 2021 increased infection rates throughout the country, especially in Ho Chi Minh City. Within a few months, the death toll rose from thirty-five to over a thousand.

2. Rossi (2017) focuses on a distinctive logic of national security, but here I am concerned with anxiety in relation to the self and everyday life.

REFERENCES

Adams, Glenn, Sara Estrada-Villalta, Daniel Sullivan, and Hazel R. Markus. 2019. The psychology of neoliberalism and the neoliberalism of psychology. *Journal of Social Issues* 75(1): 189–216.

Ahearn, Laura M. 2001. *Invitations to love: Literacy, love letters, and social change in Nepal.* Ann Arbor: University of Michigan Press.

Allison, Anne. 2013. *Precarious Japan.* Durham, NC: Duke University Press.

Anderson, Warwick. 1997. The trespass speaks: White masculinity and colonial breakdown. *The American Historical Review* 102(5): 1343–1370.

———. 2006. *Colonial pathologies: American tropical medicine, race, and hygiene in the Philippines.* Durham, NC: Duke University Press.

Appadurai, Arjun. 1996. *Modernity at large: Cultural dimensions of globalization.* Minneapolis: University of Minnesota Press.

Argenti-Pillen, Alex. 2003. *Masking trauma: How women contain violence in southern Sri Lanka.* Philadelphia: University of Pennsylvania Press.

Aries, Phillipe. 1962. *Centuries of childhood.* Robert Baldick, trans. New York: Random House.

Arsel, Zeynep, and Jonathan Y. Bean. 2013. Taste regimes and market mediated practice. *Journal of Consumer Research* 39(5): 899–917.

Aulino, Felicity. 2019. *Rituals of care: Karmic politics in an aging Thailand.* Ithaca, NY: Cornell University Press.

Barlow, David H. 2002. *Anxiety and its disorders: The nature and treatment of anxiety and panic,* 2nd edition. New York: The Guilford Press.

Bartlett, Nicholas. 2020. *Recovering histories: Life and labor after heroin in reform-era China.* Oakland: University of California Press.

Bateson, Gregory. 1958. *Naven: A survey of the problems suggested by a composite picture of the culture of a New Guinea tribe drawn from three points of view*. Palo Alto, CA: Stanford University Press.

Baxter, Amanda J., Kate M. Scott, Theo Vos, and Harvey A. Whiteford. 2013. Global prevalence of anxiety disorders: A systematic review and meta-regression. *Psychological Medicine* 43(5): 897–910.

Baxter, Amanda J., Kate M. Scott, Alize J. Ferrari, Rosanna E. Norman, Theo Vos, and Harvey A. Whiteford. 2014a. Challenging the myth of an "epidemic" of common mental disorders: Trends in the global prevalence of anxiety and depression between 1990 and 2010. *Depression and Anxiety* 31(6): 506–516.

Baxter, Amanda J., Theo Vos, Kate M. Scott, Alize J. Ferrari, and Harvey A. Whiteford. 2014b. The global burden of anxiety disorders in 2010. *Psychological Medicine* 44(11): 2363–2374.

Bayly, Susan. 2020. Beyond 'propaganda': Images and the moral citizen in late-socialist Vietnam. *Modern Asian Studies* 54(5): 1–70.

Beard, George Miller. 1881. *American nervousness, its causes and consequences: a supplement to nervous exhaustion (neurasthenia)*. New York: Putnam.

Beck, Ulrich. 1992. *Risk society: Towards a new modernity*. Mark Ritter, trans. London: Sage.

Bélanger, Daniele, Lisa B. W. Drummond, and Van Nguyen-Marshall. 2012. Who are the urban middle class in Vietnam? In *The reinvention of distinction: Modernity and the middle class in urban Vietnam*. Van Nguyen-Marshall, Lisa B. W. Drummond, and Daniele Belanger, eds. New York: Springer. Pp. 1–20.

Benedict, Ruth. 1934. Anthropology and the abnormal. *The Journal of General Psychology* 10(1): 59–82.

Beresford, Melanie. 2008. Đổi mới in review: The challenges of building market socialism in Vietnam. *Journal of Contemporary Asia* 38(2): 221–243.

Berlant, Lauren. 2011. Cruel Optimism. Durham, NC: Duke University Press.

———. 2012. *Desire/love*. Brooklyn, NY: Punctum Books.

Bhola, Poornima, and Santosh K. Chaturvedi. 2020. Neurasthenia: Tracing the journey of a protean malady. *International Review of Psychiatry* 32: 5–6, 491–499.

Bille, Mikkel, Frida Hastrup, and Tim Flohr Sørensen. 2010. An anthropology of absence. In *An anthropology of absence: Materializations of transcendence and loss*. Mikkel Bille, Friday Hastrup, and Tim Flohr Sørensen, eds. New York: Springer. Pp. 3–22.

Black, Steven P. 2018. The ethics and aesthetics of care. *Annual Review of Anthropology* 47(1): 79–95.

Bloch, Ernst. 1995. *The principle of hope*. Cambridge, MA: MIT Press.

Borovoy, Amy. 2005. *The too-good wife: Alcohol, codependency, and the politics of nurturance in postwar Japan*. Berkeley: University of California Press.

Borscheid, Peter. 1986. Romantic love or material interest: Choosing partners in nineteenth-century Germany. *Journal of Family History* 11(2): 157–168.

Bourdieu, Pierre. 1977. *Outline of a theory of practice*. Cambridge: Cambridge University Press.

———. 1984. *Distinction: A social critique of the judgment of taste*. R. Nice, trans. Cambridge, MA: Harvard University Press.

———. 2003. *Firing back: Against the tyranny of the market 2*. Loïc Wacquant, trans. London: Verso.

Bourke, Joanna. 2005. *Fear: A cultural history*. London: Virago Press.

Bradley, Mark P. 2004. Becoming *văn minh*: Civilizational discourse and visions of the self in twentieth-century Vietnam. *Journal of World History* 15(1): 65–83.

Breslau, Joshua. 2004. Cultures of trauma: Anthropological views of posttraumatic stress disorder in international health. *Culture, Medicine, and Psychiatry* 28: 113–126.

Briggs, Jean L. 1970. *Never in anger: Portrait of an Eskimo family*. Cambridge, MA: Harvard University Press.

Brook, Timothy, and Hy Van Luong. 1997. Culture and economy in the postcolonial world. In *Culture and economy: The shaping of capitalism in eastern Asia*. Timothy Brook and Hy Van Luong, eds. Ann Arbor: University of Michigan Press. Pp. 1–21.

Brown, Wendy. 2003. Neoliberalism and the end of liberal democracy. *Theory and Event* 7(1): 1–21.

Buch, Elana D. 2015. Anthropology of aging and care. *Annual Review of Anthropology* 44(1): 277–293.

Bui Thu Huong. 2010. "Let's talk about sex, baby": Sexual communication in marriage in contemporary Vietnam. *Culture, Health, and Sexuality* 12(1).

Burgess, J. Peter. 2017. For want of not: Lacan's conception of anxiety. In *Politics of Anxiety*. Emmy Eklundh, Andreja Zevnik, and Emmanuel-Pierre Guittet, eds. London: Rowman & Littlefield International. Pp. 17–36.

Cadiere, Leopold. 1957. *Croyances et pratiques religieuses de Vietnamiens, I–III*. Paris: Ecole Francaise d'Extreme-Orient.

Campbell, Brad. 2007. The making of "American": Race and nation in neurasthenic discourse. *History of Psychiatry* 18(2): 157–178.

Cherlin, Andrew J. 2004. The deinstitutionalization of American marriage. *Journal of Marriage and Family* 66(4): 848–861.

Cheung, Freda, and Keh-Ming Lin. 1997. Neurasthenia, depression and somatoform disorder in a Chinese-Vietnamese woman migrant. *Culture, Medicine and Psychiatry* 21(2): 247–258.

Chi Mai. 2022. Ngọc Bình Tâm Lý. *The Influencer*. Retrieved August 8, 2022, from https://theinfluencer-vn.translate.goog/ngoc-binh-tam-ly-song-tich-cuc-la-biet-rang-minh-se-on-du-moi-thu-xay-ra-nhu-the-nao-2595.html?_x_tr_sl=auto&_x_tr_tl=en&_x_tr_hl=en&_x_tr_pto=op,wapp.

Chin, Meejung. 2011. Family attitudes and gender role divisions of married women in contemporary Vietnam and Korea. *International Journal of Human Ecology* 12(2): 65–75.

Chua, Jocelyn Lim. 2014. *In pursuit of the good life: Aspiration and suicide in globalizing South India*. Oakland: University of California Press.

Chueng, Fanny M., Bernard W. K. Lau, and Edith Waldman. 1981. Somatization among Chinese depressives in general practice. *International Journal of Psychiatric in Medicine* 10: 361–374.

Clark, L. A. 1987. Mutual relevance off mainstream and cross-cultural psychology. *Journal of Consulting and Clinical Psychology* 55: 41–70.

Cole, Jennifer. 2010. *Sex and salvation: Imagining the future in Madagascar*. Chicago: University of Chicago Press.

Colla, Judith, Stephan Buka, David Harrington, and Jane Murphy. 2006. Depression and modernization. *Social Psychiatry and Social Epidemiology* 41(4): 271–279.

Collier, Jane Fishburne. 1997. *From duty to desire: Remaking families in a Spanish village*. Princeton, NJ: Princeton University Press.

Craciun, Mariana. 2016. The cultural work of office charisma: maintaining professional power in psychotherapy. *Theory and Society* 45: 361–383.

———. 2018. Emotions and knowledge in expert work: A comparison of two psychotherapies. *American Journal of Sociology* 123(4): 959–1003.

Craig, David. 2002. *Familiar medicine: Everyday health knowledge and practice in today's Vietnam*. Honolulu: University of Hawai'i Press.

Crapanzano, Vincent. 2004. *Imaginative horizons: An essay in literary-philosophical anthropology*. Chicago: University of Chicago Press.

Crossley, Nick. 1996. *Intersubjectivity: The fabric of social becoming*. Thousand Oaks, CA: Sage.

Csordas, Thomas J. 1990. Embodiment as a Paradigm for Anthropology. *Ethos* 18: 5–47.

———. 1993. Somatic Modes of Attention. *Cultural Anthropology* 8: 135–156.

———. 1994. Self and person. In *Handbook of psychological anthropology*. Phillip Bock, ed. Westport, CT: Greenwood. Pp. 331–350.

———. 2008. Intersubjectivity and intercorporeality. *Subjectivity* 22: 110–121.

Csordas, Thomas J., Christopher Dole, Allen L. Tran, Matthew Strickland, and Michael G. Storck. 2010. Ways of asking, ways of telling. *Culture, Medicine, and Psychiatry* 34: 29–55.

Daniel, E. Valentine. 1996. *Charred lullabies: Chapters in an anthropography of violence*. Princeton, NJ: Princeton University Press.

Dao, Amy. 2020. What it means to say "I don't have any money to buy health insurance" in rural Vietnam: How anticipatory activities shape health insurance enrollment. *Social Science and Medicine* 266: 113335.

Đào Duy Anh. 1932. *Hán-Việt từ điển giản yếu* [*Sino-Vietnamese Dictionary*]. Hanoi: NXB Văn hóa Thông tin [Culture and Information Press].

Das, Veena, and Arthur Kleinman. 2000. Introduction. In *Violence and Subjectivity*. V. Das, A. Kleinman, M. Ramphele, and P. Reynolds, eds. Berkeley: University of California Press. Pp. 1–18.

Das, Veena, Arthur Kleinman, Mamphela Ramphele, and Pamela Reynolds, eds. 2000. *Violence and subjectivity*. Berkeley: University of California Press.

Davis, Coralynn V. 2014. Transnational marriage: Modern imaginings, relational realignments, and persistent inequalities. *Ethnos* 79(5): 585–609.

Dere, Jessica, Jiahong Sun, Yue Zhao, Tonje Persson, Xiongzhao Zhu, Shuqiao Yao, R. Michael Bagby, and Andrew G. Ryder. 2013. Beyond "somatization" and "psychologization": Symptom-level variation in depressed Han Chinese and Euro-Canadian outpatients. *Frontiers in Psychology* 4: 377.

Desjarlais, Robert R. 1992. *Body and emotion: The aesthetics of illness and healing in the Nepal Himalayas*. Philadelphia: University of Pennsylvania Press.

Diệu Nguyên. 2013. Chăm lo sức khoẻ tâm thần. *Tuổi Trẻ*. http://tuoitre.vn/tin/song-khoe/20130625/cham-lo-suc-khoe-tam-than/555722.html, accessed 6/15/15.

Dixon, Thomas. 2012. "Emotion": The history of a key word in crisis. *Emotion Review* 4(4): 338–344.

Drummond, Lisa W. 2000. Street scenes: Practices of public and private space in urban Vietnam. *Urban Studies* 37(12): 2377–2391.

———. 2012. Middle class landscapes in a transforming city: Hanoi in the 21st century. In *The reinvention of distinction: Modernity and the middle class in urban Vietnam*. Van

Nguyen-Marshall, Lisa Welch Drummond, and Melanie Belanger, eds. Singapore: Asia Research Institute. Pp. 79–94.

Duncan, Whitney L. 2017. Psicoeducación in the land of magical thoughts: Culture and mental health practice in a changing Oaxaca. *American Ethnologist* 44(1): 36–51.

———. 2018. *Transforming therapy: Mental health practice and cultural change in Mexico.* Nashville, TN: Vanderbilt University Press.

Duong Anh Vuong, Ewout Van Ginnekin, Son Thai Ha, and Reinhard Busse. 2011. Mental health in Vietnam: Burden of disease and availability of services. *Asian Journal of Psychiatry* 4(1): 65–70.

Dương Liễu. 2017. "3,6 Triệu Người Việt Nam Mắc Chứng Trầm Cảm." *Tuoi Tre Online.* April 7, 2017. http://tuoitre.vn/news-1293822.htm.

Earl, Catherine. 2014a. "Life as lived and life as talked about": Family, love, and marriage in twenty-first century Vietnam. In *Routledge Handbook of Sexuality Studies in East Asia.* Mark McClelland and Vera Mackie, eds. New York: Routledge. Pp. 101–111.

———. 2014b. *Vietnam's new middle classes: Gender, career, city.* Copenhagen: NIAS Press.

———. 2020. Future-making tactics: Exploring middle-class living and green practices in Ho Chi Minh City, Vietnam. *Ethnos* 85(3): 454–470.

Ecks, Stefan. 2016. Commentary: Ethnographic critiques of global mental health. *Transcultural Psychiatry* 53(6): 804–808.

Edington, Claire E. 2019. *Beyond the asylum: Mental illness in French colonial Vietnam.* Ithaca, NY: Cornell University Press.

———. 2021. The most social of maladies: Rethinking the history of psychiatry from the edges of empire. *Culture, Medicine, and Psychiatry* 45: 343–358.

Eklundh, Emmy, Emmanuel-Pierre Guittet, and Andreja Zevnik. 2017. Introduction: The politics of anxiety. In *Politics of Anxiety.* Emmy Eklundh, Andreja Zevnik, and Emmanuel-Pierre Guittet, eds. London: Rowman & Littlefield International. Pp. 1–14.

Elinoff, Eli A. 2012. Smouldering aspirations: Burning buildings and the politics of belonging in contemporary Isan. *Journal of Southeast Asia Research* 20(3): 381–398.

Escobar, Arturo. 1991. Anthropology and the development encounter: The making and marketing of development anthropology. *American Ethnologist* 18: 658–682.

Ewing, Katherine P. 1990. The illusion of wholeness: Culture, self, and the experience of inconsistency. *Ethos* 18(3): 251–278.

Fabrega, H. 1990. Hispanic mental health research: A case for cultural psychiatry. *Hispanic Journal of Behavioral Science* 12: 339–365.

Farrer, James. 2002. *Opening up: Youth sex culture and market reform in Shanghai.* Chicago: University of Chicago Press.

Fassin, Didier, and Richard Rechtman. 2009. *The empire of trauma: An inquiry into the condition of victimhood.* Princeton, NJ: Princeton University Press.

Fisher, Jane, Thach Tran, Buoi Thi La, Kelsi Kriitmaa, Doreen Rosenthal, and Tuan Tran. 2010. Common perimental mental disorders in northern Vietnam: Community prevalence and health care use. *Bulletin of the World Health Organization* 88: 737–745.

Foucault, Michel. 1988. *Technologies of the self: A seminar with Michel Foucault.* Luther H. Martin, Hugh Gutman, and Patrick W. Hutton, eds. Boston: University of Massachusetts Press.

Freeman, Carla. 2007. Neoliberalism and the marriage of reputation and respectability: Entrepreneurship and the Barbadian middle class. In *Love and globalization: Transformations of intimacy in the contemporary world.* M. B. Padilla, J. S. Hirsch, M. Muñoz-Laboy, R. Sember, and R. G. Parker, eds. Nashville, TN: Vanderbilt University Press. Pp. 3–37.

———. 2011. Neoliberalism: Embodying and affecting neoliberalism. In *A companion to the anthropology of the body and embodiment.* Frances E. Mascia-Lees, ed. New York: Blackwell. Pp. 353–369.

———. 2014. *Entrepreneurial selves: Neoliberal respectability and the making of a Caribbean middle class.* Durham, NC: Duke University Press.

Freud, Sigmund. 1919 (2003). *The uncanny.* New York: Penguin Modern Classics.

———. 1936. Inhibitions, symptoms and anxiety. *The Psychoanalytic Quarterly* 5(1): 1–28.

Friedman, Sara L. 2005. The intimacy of state power: Marriage, liberation, and socialist subjects in southeastern China. *American Ethnologist* 32(2): 312–327.

Fromm, Erich. 1941. *Escape from freedom.* New York: Farrar & Rinehart.

Furedi, Frank. 2004. *Therapy culture: Cultivating vulnerability in an uncertain age.* London: Routledge.

Gammeltoft, Tine M. 1999. *Women's bodies, women's worries: Health and family planning in a Vietnamese rural commune.* Richmond, UK: Curzon.

———. 2014a. *Haunting images: A cultural account of selective reproduction in Vietnam.* Oakland: University of California Press.

———. 2014b. Toward an anthropology of the imaginary: Specters of disability in Vietnam. *Ethos* 42(2): 153–174.

———. 2018. Belonging: Comprehending subjectivity in Vietnam and beyond. *Social Analysis* 62(1): 76–95.

———. 2021. Spectral kinship: Understanding how Vietnamese women endure domestic distress. *American Ethnologist* 48(1): 22–36.

Garcia, Angela. 2010. *The pastoral clinic: Addiction and dispossession along the Rio Grande.* Berkeley: University of California Press.

Garro, Linda C. 2003. Narrating troubling experiences. *Transcultural Psychiatry* 40(1): 5–43.

Geertz, Clifford. 1979. From the native's point of view: On the nature of anthropological understanding. In *Interpretive social science: A second look.* Paul Rabinow and William M. Sullivan, eds. Berkeley: University of California Press. Pp. 225–242.

Geurts, Kathryn L. 2002. *Culture and the senses: Bodily ways of knowing in an African community.* Berkeley: University of California Press.

Giddens, Anthony. 1991. *Modernity and self-identity: Self and society in the late modern age.* Stanford, CA: Stanford University Press.

———. 1993. *The transformation of intimacy: Sexuality, love, and eroticism in modern societies.* Palo Alto, CA: Stanford University Press.

Gold, Steven. 1992. Mental health and illness in Vietnamese refugees. *Journal of Medicine* 157(3): 290–294.

Good, Byron J., and Arthur M. Kleinman. 2019. Culture and anxiety: Cross-cultural evidence for the patterning of anxiety disorders. In *Anxiety and the anxiety disorders.* A. H. Tuma and J. D. Maser, eds. New York: Routledge. Pp. 297–324.

Goode, William J. 1959. The theoretical importance of love. *American Sociological Review* 24(1): 38–47.

Goodkind, Daniel. 1996. State agendas, local sentiments: Vietnamese wedding practices amidst socialist transformations. *Social Forces* 75(2): 717–742.

Gould, Deborah B. 2009. *Moving politics: Emotion and ACT UP's fight against AIDS.* Chicago: University of Chicago Press.

Greenhalgh, Susan, and Edwin Winckler. 2005. *Governing China's population: From Leninist to neoliberal biopolitics.* Stanford, CA: Stanford University Press.

Guarnaccia, Peter J., Roberto Lewis-Fernandez, and Melissa Rivera Marano. 2003. Toward a Puerto Rican popular nosology: *Nervios* and *Ataque de nervios. Culture, Medicine, and Psychiatry* 27(3): 339–366.

Hansen, Arve. 2017. Consuming *doi moi:* Development and middle class consumption in Vietnam. *Journal of Social Sciences and Humanities* 3(2): 171–186.

Harms, Erik. 2009. Vietnam's civilizing process and the retreat from the street: A turtle's eye view. *City & Society* 21(2): 182–206.

———. 2011. *Saigon's edge: On the margins of Ho Chi Minh City.* Minneapolis: University of Minnesota Press.

Harpham, Trudy. 1994. Urbanization and mental health in developing countries: A research role for social scientists, public health professionals and social psychiatrists. *Social Science and Medicine* 39(2): 233–245.

Harvey, David. 2007. *A brief history of neoliberalism.* Oxford: Oxford University Press.

Hays, Pamela A. 2009. Integrating evidence-based practice, cognitive-behavior therapy, and multicultural therapy: Ten steps for culturally competent practice. *Professional Psychology: Research and Practice* 40(4): 354–360.

Hệ thống chăm sóc sức khoẻ tâm thần cộng đồng tại Thành Phố Hồ Chí Minh [Community mental health care system in Ho Chi Minh City]. 2007. Retrieved January 10, 2012 from http://www.bvtt-tphcm.org.vn/gioi-thieu-benh-vien/210-h-thng-chm-soc-sc-khe-tam-thn-cng-ng-ti-tp-h-chi-minh.html.

Heidegger, Martin. 1962. *Being and time.* New York: Harper & Row.

Heiman, Rachel, Mark Liechty, and Carla Freeman. 2012. Introduction: Charting an anthropology of the middle classes. In *The global middle classes: Theorizing through ethnography.* Rachel Heiman, Carla Freeman, and Mark Leichty, eds. Santa Fe, NM: School for Advanced Research Press. Pp. 3–30.

Hien, Nina. 2012. Ho Chi Minh City's beauty regime: Haptic technologies of the self in the new millenium. *Positions* 20(2): 473–493.

Higgins, Rylan G. 2008. Negotiating the middle: Interactions of class, gender, and consumerism among the middle-class in Ho Chi Minh City, Vietnam. Doctoral dissertation, University of Arizona. ProQuest Dissertations Publishing.

Hinton, Devon, Dara Cheean, Vuth Pich, Stefan Hofmann, and David Barlow. 2006. Tinnitus among Cambodians: Relationship to PTSD severity. *Journal of Traumatic Stress* 19(4): 541–546.

Hinton, Devon, and Byron Good, eds. 2009. *Culture and panic disorder.* Palo Alto, CA: Stanford University Press.

Hinton, Devon, Ladson Hinton, Minh Tran, Men Nguyen, Lim Nguyen, Curtis Hsia, and Mark H. Pollack. 2007. Orthostatic panic attacks among Vietnamese refugees. *Transcultural Psychiatry* 44(4): 515–544.

Hinton, Devon, and Susan Hinton. 2002. Panic disorder, somatization, and the new cross-cultural psychiatry: The seven bodies of a medical anthropology of panic. *Culture, Medicine, and Psychiatry* 26: 155–178.

Hinton, Devon, Susan Hinton, Thang Pham, Ha Chau, and Minh Tran. 2003. "Hit by the wind" and temperature shift panic among Vietnamese refugees. *Transcultural Psychiatry* 49(3): 342–376.

Hinton, Devon, and Roberto Lewis-Fernandez. 2010. Idioms of distress among trauma survivors: Subtypes and clinical utility. *Culture, Medicine, and Psychiatry* 34: 209–218.

Hinton, Devon, Vuth Pich, Dara Chhean, and Mark H. Pollack. 2004. Olfactory panic among Cambodian refugees: A contextual approach. *Transcultural Psychiatry* 4(2): 155–199.

Hinton, Devon, Ria Reis, and Joop de Jong. 2015. The "thinking a lot" idiom of distress and PTSD: An examination of their relationship among traumatized Cambodian refugees using the "Thinking a lot" questionnaire. *Medical Anthropology Quarterly* 29(3): 357–380.

Hirsch, Jennifer S., and Holly Wardlow, eds. 2006. *Modern loves: The anthropology of romantic courtship and companionate marriage.* Ann Arbor: University of Michigan Press.

Hirschman, Charles, and Nguyen Huu Minh. 2002. Tradition and change in Vietnamese family structure in the Red River Delta. *Journal of Marriage and Family* 64: 1063–1079.

Hoài Thanh and Hoài Chân. 1988 (1942). *Thi nhân Việt Nam, 1932–1941.* Hanoi: NXB Văn học.

Hoang, Kimberly K. 2015. *Dealing in desire: Asian ascendancy, Western decline, and the hidden currencies of global sex work.* Oakland: University of California Press.

Hoblyn, Jennifer C., Steve L. Balt, Stephanie A. Woodward, and John O. Brooks III. 2009. Substance use disorders as risk factors for psychiatric hospitalization in bipolar disorder. *Psychiatric Service* 60(1): 50–55.

Hochschild, Arlie R. 1983. *The managed heart: Commercialization of human feeling.* Berkeley: University of California Press.

Hodgetts, Darrin, and Ottilie Stolte. 2017. *Urban poverty and health inequalities: A relational approach.* New York: Routledge.

Hollan, Douglas W. 2001. Developments in person-centered ethnography. In *The psychology of cultural experience.* Carmella C. Moore and Holly F. Mathews, eds. Cambridge: Cambridge University Press. Pp. 48–67.

Hollan, Douglas W., and C. Jason Throop, eds. 2011. *The anthropology of empathy: Experiencing the lives of others in Pacific societies.* Brooklyn, NY: Berghahn Books

Hopper, Kim. 2007. Rethinking social recovery in schizophrenia: What a capabilities approach might offer. *Social Science and Medicine* 65(5): 868–879.

Horton, Paul, and Helle Rydstrøm. 2011. Heterosexual masculinity in contemporary Vietnam: Privileges, power, and protest. *Men and Masculinities* 14(5): 542–564.

Horwitz, Allan V. 2010. How an age of anxiety became an age of depression. *The Milbank Quarterly* 88(1): 112–138.

———. 2013. *Anxiety: A short history.* Baltimore: Johns Hopkins University Press.

Horwitz, Allan, and Jerome Wakefield. 2012. *All we have to fear: Psychiatry's transformation of natural anxieties into mental disorders.* Oxford: Oxford University Press.

Huang, Hsuan-yin. 2014. The emergence of the psycho-boom in contemporary urban China. In *Psychiatry and Chinese history.* H. Chiang, ed. London: Pickering & Chatto. Pp. 183–204.

———. 2015. From psychotherapy to psycho-boom: A historical overview of psychotherapy in China. *Psychoanalysis and Psychotherapy in China* 1: 1–30.

Husserl, Edmund. 1999. *Cartesian meditations: An introduction to phenomenology*. Dorion Cairns, trans. Dordrecht, The Netherlands: Kluwer Academic Press.

Hwang, Wie-Chin, Jeffrey J. Wood, Keh-Ming Lin, and Freda Cheung. 2006. Cognitive-behavioral therapy with Chinese Americans: Research, theory, and clinical practice. *Cognitive and Behavioral Practice* 13(4): 293–303.

Illouz, Eva. 1997. Introduction to the sociology of love. In *Consuming the romantic utopia: Love and the cultural contradictions of capitalism*. Berkeley: University of California Press. Pp. 1–22.

———. 2007. *Cold intimacies: The making of emotional capitalism*. Cambridge: Polity Press.

———. 2008. *Saving the modern soul: Therapy, emotions, and the culture of self-help*. Berkeley: University of California Press.

———. 2012. *Why love hurts: A sociological explanation*. New York: Polity Press.

Iwamasa, Gayle Y., Curtis Hsia, and Devon Hinton. 2019. Cognitive behavior therapy with Asian Americans. In *Culturally responsive cognitive behavior therapy: Practice and supervision*. Gayle Y. Iwamasa and Pamela A. Hays, eds. American Psychological Association. Pp. 129–159.

Jackson, Peter, and Jonathan Everts. 2010. Anxiety as social practice. *Environment and Planning* 42: 2791–2806.

Jamieson, Neil. 1995. *Understanding Vietnam*. Berkeley: University of California Press.

Jankowiak, William R., and Edward F. Fischer. 1992. A cross-cultural perspective on romantic love. *Ethnology* 31(2): 129–155.

Jellema, Kate. 2005. Making good on debt: The remoralixation of wealth in post-revolutionary Vietnam. *Asia Pacific Journal of Anthropology* 6(3): 231–248.

Jenkins, Janis H. 1991. The state construction of affect: Political ethos and mental health among Salvadoran refugees. *Culture, Medicine, and Psychiatry* 15(2): 139–165.

———. 1994. The psychocultural study of emotion and mental disorder. In *Handbook of psychological anthropology*. Phillip Bock, ed. Westport, CT: Greenwood. Pp. 97–120.

Jenkins, Janis H., and Robert Barrett. 2004. Introduction. In *Schizophrenia, culture, and subjectivity*. Janis H. Jenkins and Robert Barrett, eds. Cambridge: Cambridge University Press. Pp. 1–25.

Jenkins, Janis H., and Norma Cofresi. 1998. The sociosomatic course of depression and trauma: A cultural analysis of suffering and resilience in the life of a Puerto Rican woman. *Psychosomatic Medicine* 60(4): 439–447.

Jenkins, Janis H., and Marta Valiente. 1994. Bodily transactions of the passions: *El calor* among Salvadoran women refugees. In *Embodiment and experience: The existential ground of culture and self*. Thomas J. Csordas, ed. Cambridge: Cambridge University Press.

Jones, Carla. 2004 Whose stress? Emotion work in middle-class Javanese homes. *Ethnos* 69(4): 509–528.

Kelley, Liam C. 2006. "Confucianism" in Vietnam: A state of the field essay. *Journal of Vietnamese Studies* 1(1–2): 314–370.

Kierkegaard, Søren. 1844 (2014). *The concept of dread: A simple psychologically oriented deliberation in view of the dogmatic problem of hereditary sin*. Alistar Hannay, trans. New York: Liveright.

King, Victor T., Phuong An Nguyen, and Nguyen Huu Minh. 2008. Professional middle class youth in post-reform Vietnam: Identity, continuity and change. *Modern Asian Studies* 42(4): 783–813.

Kipnis, Andrew. 2012. Introduction: Chinese modernity and the individual psyche. In *Chinese modernity and the individual psyche*. Andrew B. Kipnis, ed. New York: Palgrave Macmillan. Pp. 1–18.

Kirmayer, Laurence J. 2006. Culture and psychotherapy in a creolizing world. *Transcultural Psychiatry* 43(2): 163–168.

———. 2007. Psychotherapy and the cultural concept of the person. *Transcultural Psychiatry* 44(2): 232–257.

Kirmayer, Laurence J., and Eugene Raikhel. 2009. From Amrita to Substance D: Psychopharmacology, political economy, and technologies of the self. *Transcultural Psychiatry* 46(1): 5–15.

Kitanaka, Junko. 2011. *Depression in Japan: Psychiatric cures for a society in distress*. Princeton, NJ: Princeton University Press.

———. 2012. *Depression in Japan: Psychiatric cures for a nation in distress*. Princeton, NJ: Princeton University Press.

Klein, Melanie. 1948. A contribution to the theory of anxiety and guilt. *International Journal of Psychoanalysis* 29: 114–123.

Kleinman, Arthur. 1982. Neurasthenia and depression: A study of somatization and culture in China. *Culture, Medicine, and Psychiatry* 6: 117–190.

———. 1986. *Social origins of distress and disease: Depression, neurasthenia, and pain in modern China*. New Haven, CT: Yale University Press.

———. 2000. The violence of everyday life: The multiple forms and dynamics of social violence. In *Violence and subjectivity*. Veena Das, Arthur Kleinman, Mamphela Ramphele, and Pamela Reynolds, eds. Berkeley: University of California Press. Pp. 226–241.

———. 2010. Remaking the moral person: Implications for health. *The Lancet* 375(9720): 1074–1075.

Kleinman, Arthur, Veena Das, and Margaret Lock, eds. 1997. *Social suffering*. Berkeley: University of California Press.

Kleinman, Arthur, and Joan Kleinman. 1991. Suffering and its professional transformation: Towards an ethnography of interpersonal experience. *Culture, Medicine, and Psychiatry* 15(3): 275–301.

Krakauer, Jon. 1996. *Into the wild*. New York: Random House.

Kristeva, Julia. 1982. *Powers of horror: An essay in abjection*. Leon S. Roudiez, trans. New York: Columbia University Press.

Kwiatkowski, Lynn. 2016. Domestic violence and the "happy family" in northern Vietnam. *Anthropology Now* 3: 20–28.

Kwon, Heonik. 2008. *Ghosts of war in Vietnam*. Cambridge: Cambridge University Press.

Lacan, Jacques. 2016. *Anxiety: The seminar of Jacques Lacan*. A. R. Price, trans. New York: Polity.

Laidlaw, James. 2002. For an anthropology of ethics and freedom. *Journal of the Royal Anthropological Institute* 8(2): 311–332.

Lakoff, George, and Mark Johnson. 1980. *Metaphors we live by*. Chicago: University of Chicago Press.

Lam, Andrew. 2005. Stress—A new word for a new Vietnam. *New American Media*. http://news.newamericamedia.org/news/view_article.html?article_id=d79d88c7a7b74f4e5346b613939c59f5 (accessed July 12, 2014).

Lee, Haiyan. 2007. *Revolution of the heart: A genealogy of love in China, 1900–1950*. Stanford, CA: Stanford University Press.

Lee, Sing. 2011. Depression: Coming of age in China. In *Deep China: The moral life of the person, what anthropology and psychiatry tell us about China today*. A. Kleinman, Y. Yan, J. Sun, S. Lee, E. Zhang, P. Tianshu, W. Fei, and G. Jinhua, eds. Berkeley: University of California Press. Pp. 177–212.

Lerner, Julia, and Michelle Rivkin-Fish. 2021. On emotionalisation of public domains. *Emotions and Society* 3(1): 3–14.

Leshkowich, Ann Marie. 2006. Woman, Buddhist, entrepreneur: Gender, moral values, and class anxiety in late socialist Vietnam. *Journal of Vietnamese Studies* 1(1–2): 277–313.

———. 2012. Finances, family, fashion, fitness…and freedom? The changing lives of urban middle-class Vietnamese women. In *The reinvention of distinction: Modernity and the middle class in urban Vietnam*. Van Nguyen-Marshall, Lisa Welch Drummond, and Melanie Belanger, eds. Singapore: Asia Research Institute.

———. 2014a. *Essential trade: Vietnam women in a changing marketplace*. Honolulu: University of Hawai'i Press.

———. 2014b. Standardized forms of Vietnamese selfhood: An ethnographic genealogy of documentation. *American Ethnologist* 41(1): 143–162.

———. 2022. Market personhood in urban southern Vietnam. In *Routledge handbook of contemporary Vietnam*. Jonathan D. London, ed. London: Routledge.

Leshkowich, Ann Marie, and Kirsten Endres. 2018. Space, mobility, borders, and trading frictions. In *Traders in motion: Identities and contestations in the Vietnamese marketplace*. Ithaca, NY: Cornell University Press. Pp. 1–16.

Leshkowich, Ann Marie, and Carla Jones. 2003. What happens when Asian chic becomes chic in Asia? *Fashion Theory* 7(3): 281–300.

Lester, Rebecca J. 2013. Back from the edge of existence: A critical anthropology of trauma. *Transcultural Psychiatry* 50(5): 753–762.

Levy, Robert. 1984. Emotion, knowing, and culture. In *Culture theory: Essays on mind, self, and emotion*. Richard Shweder and Robert LeVine, eds. Cambridge: Cambridge University Press. Pp. 214–237.

Levy, Robert I., and Douglas W. Hollan. 1988. Person-centered interviewing and observation in anthropology. In *Handbook of methods in cultural anthropology*. H. Russel Bernard, ed. Walnut Creek, CA: Altamira Press. Pp. 333–364.

Liên Châu. 2017. "Mỗi Năm Có Khoảng 40.000 Người Tự Sát Do Trầm Cảm" [40,000 People Commit Suicide Due to Depression]. *Báo Thanh Niên*. April 5, 2017. https://thanhnien.vn/content/NjUoNzc4.html.

Lifton, Robert Jay. 1999. *The protean self: Human resilience in an age of fragmentation*. Chicago: University of Chicago Press.

Lindholm, Charles. 1998. Love and structure. *Theory, Culture, and Society* 15(3–4): 243–263.

Lindquist, Johan. 2008. *The anxieties of mobility: Migration and tourism in the Indonesian borderlands*. Honolulu: University of Hawai'i Press.

Lipset, David. 2004. Modernity without romance? Masculinity and desire in courtship stories told by young papua new guinean men. *American Ethnologist* 31(2): 205–224.

Liu, Xin. 2002. *The otherness of self: A genealogy of the self in contemporary China*. Ann Arbor: University of Michigan Press.

Lloyd, Stephanie, and Nicolas Moreau. 2011. Pursuit of a 'normal life': Mood, anxiety, and their disordering. *Medical Anthropology* 30(6): 591–609.

Lock, Margaret. 1987. Protests of a good wife and wise mother: The medicalization of distress in Japan. In *Health, illness, and medical care in Japan: Cultural and social dimensions*. Edward Norbeck and Margaret Lock, eds. Honolulu: University of Hawai'i Press. Pp. 130–157.

Lopez, Steven Regeser, and Peter J. J. Guarnaccia. 2000. Cultural psychopathology: Uncovering the social world of mental illness. *Annual Review of Psychology* 51: 571–598.

Low, Setha. 1985. Culturally interpreted symptoms or culture-bound syndromes: A cross-cultural review of nerves. *Social Science and Medicine* 21(2): 187–196.

Lund, Crick, Carrie Brooke-Summer, Florence Baingana, Emily Claire Baron, Erica Breuer, Prabha Chandra, Johannes Haushofer, Helen Herrman, Mark Jordans, Christian Kieling, Maria Elena Medinca-Mora, Ellen Morgan, et al. 2018. Social determinants of mental disorders and the sustainable development goals: A systematic review of reviews. *The Lancet Psychiatry* 5(4): 357–369.

Luong, Hy Van. 1984. "Brother" and "uncle": An analysis of rules, structural contradictions, and meaning in Vietnamese kinship. *American Anthropologist* 86(2): 290–315.

———. 1989. Vietnamese kinship: Structuralist principles and the socialist transformation in Northern Vietnam. *Journal of Asian Studies* 48(4): 741–756.

Luthra, A., and Simon Wessely. 2004. Unloading the trunk: Neurasthenia, CFS, and race. *Social Science and Medicine* 58(11): 2363–2369.

Lutz, Catherine A. 1982. The domain of emotion words on Ifaluk. *American Ethnologist* 9 (1): 113–128.

———. 1988. *Unnatural emotions: Everyday sentiments on a Micronesian atoll and their challenge to Western theory.* Chicago: University of Chicago Press.

Lutz, Catherine A., and Lila Abu-Lughod, eds. 1990. *Language and the politics of emotion.* Cambridge: Cambridge University Press.

Lutz, Tom. 1991. *American nervousness, 1903: An anecdotal history.* Ithaca, NY: Cornell University Press.

Ma, Zhiying. 2012. Psychiatric subjectivity and cultural resistance: Experience and explanations of schizophrenia in contemporary China. In *Chinese modernity and the individual psyche*. Andrew Kipnis, ed. New York: Palgrave Macmillan. Pp. 203–227.

MacLean, Ken. 2008. The rehabilitation of an uncomfortable past: Everyday life in Vietnam during the subsidy period (1975–1986). *History and Anthropology* 19(3): 281–303.

Makovicky, Nicolette. 2014. Me, Inc.? Untangling neoliberalism, personhood, and postsocialism. In *Neoliberalism, personhood, and postsocialism: Enterprising selves in changing economies*. Nicolette Makovicky, ed. Furnham, UK: Ashgate. Pp. 1–16.

Marr, David G. 2000. Concepts of "individual" and "self" in twentieth-century Vietnam. *Modern Asian Studies* 34(3): 769–796.

———. 2003. A passion for modernity: Intellectuals and the media. In *Postwar Vietnam: Dynamics of a transforming society*. Hy Van Luong, ed. Lanham, MD: Rowman and Littlefield. Pp. 257–295.

Marsella, Anthony. 1998. Urbanization, mental health, and social deviancy: A review of issues and research. *American Psychologist* 53(6): 624–634.

Maslow, Abraham H. 1943. A theory of human motivation. *Psychological Review* 50(4): 370–396.

Massumi, Brian. 2010. The future birth of the affective fact: The political ontology of threat. In *The affect theory reader*. Melissa Gregg and Gregory J. Seigworth, eds. Durham, NC: Duke University Press. Pp. 52–70.

Mattingly, Cheryl. 2010. *The paradox of hope: Journeys through a clinical borderland.* Berkeley: University of California Press.

———. 2014. *Moral laboratories: Family peril and the struggle for a good life.* Oakland: University of California Press.

Mattingly, Cheryl, and C. Jason Throop. 2018. The anthropology of ethics and morality. *Annual Review of Anthropology* 47(1): 475–492.

Matza, Tomas. 2018. *Shock therapy: Psychology, precarity, and well-being in postsocialist Russia.* Durham, NC: Duke University Press.

Mauss, Marcel. 1990 (1950). *The gift: The form and reason for exchange in archaic societies.* New York: W.W. Norton.

May, Rollo. 1950. *The meaning of anxiety.* New York: W.W. Norton.

McElwee, Pamela D. 2005. "There is nothing that is difficult": History and hardship on and after the Ho Chi Minh Trail in North Vietnam. *The Asia Pacific Journal of Anthropology* 6(3): 197–215.

McGrath, Jason. 2008. *Postsocialist modernity: Chinese cinema, literature, and criticism in the market age.* Stanford, CA: Stanford University Press.

McHale, Shawn. 1995. Printing and power: Vietnamese debates over women's place in society, 1918–1934. In *Essays into Vietnamese pasts.* Keith Taylor and John Whitmore, eds. Ithaca, NY: Cornell Southeast Asia Program. Pp. 173–194.

———. 2004. *Print and power: Confucianism, communism, Buddhism, and the making of modern Vietnam.* Honolulu: University of Hawai'i Press.

McMullin, Juliet, and Amy Dao. 2014. Watching as an ordinary affect: Care and mothers' preemption of injury in child supervision. *Subjectivity* 7: 171–189.

Middleton, Townsend. 2013. Anxious belongings: Anxiety and the politics of belonging in subnationalist Darjeeling. *American Anthropologist* 115(4): 608–621.

Ministry of Health. 2002. National epidemiology of mental disorders. Unpublished report by Federal Psychiatric Hospital I submitted to the World Health Organization.

Monnais, Laurence. 2012. Colonised and neurasthenic: From the appropriation of a word to the reality of a malaise de civlisation in urban French Vietnam. *Health and History* 14(1): 121–142.

Monnais, Laurence, C. Michelle Thompson, and Ayo Wahlberg. 2012. Introduction: Southern medicine for southern people. In *Southern medicine for southern people: Vietnamese medicine in the making.* Laurence Monnais, C. Michelle Thompson, and Ayo Wahlberg, eds. Cambridge: Cambridge Scholars. Pp. 1–16.

Mozzarella, William. 2009. Affect: What is it good for? In *Enchantments of modernity: Empire, nation, globalization.* Saurabh Dube, ed. London: Routledge.

Myers, Neely, Rebecca Lester, and Kim Hopper. 2016. Reflections on the anthropology of public psychiatry: The potential and limitations of transdisciplinary work. *Transcultural Psychiatry* 53(4): 419–426.

Nash, Jesse W., and Elizabeth Trinh Nguyen. 1995. *Romance, gender, and region in a Vietnamese-American community: Tales of God and beautiful women*. Lewiston, NY: Edwin Mellen Press.

Nations, Marilyn, Linda Camino, and Frederick Walker. 1988. Nerves: Folk idiom for anxiety and depression? *Social Science and Medicine* 26(12): 1245–1259.

Nelson, Alex J., and William Jankowiak. 2021. Love's ethnographic record: Beyond the love/arranged marriage dichotomy and other false essentialisms. In *International handbook of love: Transcultural and transdisciplinary perspectives*. Claude-Hélène Mayer and Elisabeth Vanderheiden, eds. New York: Springer. Pp. 41–58.

Neocleous, Mark. 2017. Anxiety: Trauma: Resilience. In *Politics of anxiety*. Emmy Eklundh, Andreja Zevnik, and Emmanuel-Pierre Guittet, eds. London: Rowman & Littlefield International. Pp. 61–78.

Ng, Emily. 2009. Headache of the state, enemy of the self: Bipolar disorder and cultural change in urban China. *Culture, Medicine, and Psychiatry* 33: 421–450.

Ngai, Sianne. 2007. *Ugly feelings*. Cambridge, MA: Harvard University Press.

Ngọc Bình [@ngocbinhtamly]. March 19, 2021. "Bạn căng thẳng sau một tuần? DÀNH CHO BẠN!" https://www.tiktok.com/@ngocbinhtamly/video/6941351678897622273?is_from_webapp=1&sender_device=pc&web_id=7128865888747324974.

———. June 10, 2021. "Mình chỉ muốn nói là trên tiktok còn rất nhiều người sẵn sàng cho b những lời khuyên bổ ích." https://www.tiktok.com/@ngocbinhtamly/video/69723 88573060320514?is_from_webapp=1&sender_device=pc&web_id=7128865888747 324974.

Nguyen, Dat Manh. 2020. Unburdening the heart: Urban therapeutic Buddhism and youth well-being in Hồ Chí Minh City. *Journal of Vietnamese Studies* 15(4): 63–98.

Nguyen, Hoa Nga, and Pranee Liamputtong. 2007. Sex, love, and gender norms: Sexual life and experience of a group of young people in Ho Chi Minh City, Vietnam. *Sexual Health* 4(1): 63–69.

Nguyen, Phuong An. 2007. "Relationships based on love and relationships based on needs": Emerging trends in youth sex culture in contemporary urban Vietnam. *Modern Asian Studies* 41: 287–313.

Nguyễn, Thịnh, Janette Brooks, Jacqueline Frayne, Felice Watt, and Jane Fisher. 2015. The preconception needs of women with severe mental illness: A consecutive clinical case series. *Journal of Psychosomatic Obstetrics and Gynecology* 36(3): 87–93.

Nguyen, Viet Thanh. 2016. *Nothing ever dies: Vietnam and the memory of war*. Cambridge, MA: Harvard University Press.

Nguyen-Marshall, Van, Lisa Welch Drummond, and Daniele Bélanger, eds. 2012. *The reinvention of distinction: Modernity and the middle class in urban Vietnam*. London: Springer Dordrecht Heidelberg.

Nguyễn Ngọc Quang. 2004. Đặc điểm lâm sàng rối loạn trầm cảm và lo âu ở bệnh nhân AIDS (Clinical characteristics of depressive and anxiety disorders in patients with AIDS). *Chuyện Đề Tâm Thần Học (Issues in Psychiatry)* 3: 7–12.

Nguyen Tu, Thuy Linh. 2021. *Experiments in skin: Race and beauty in the shadows of Vietnam*. Durham, NC: Duke University Press.

Nguyễn-Võ Thu-Hương. 2006. The body wager: Materialist resignification of Vietnamese women workers. *Gender, Place & Culture* 13(3): 267–281.

————. 2008. *The ironies of freedom: Sex, culture, and neoliberal governance in Vietnam.* Seattle: University of Washington Press.

Nichter, Mark. 2010. Idioms of distress revisited. *Culture, Medicine, and Psychiatry* 34: 401–416.

Niemi, Marie E., T. Falkenberg, Mai T. T. Nguyen, Minh T. N. Nguyen, Vikram Patel, and Elizabeth Faxelid. 2009. The social contexts of depression during motherhood: A study of explanatory models in Vietnam. *Journal of Affective Disorders* 124 (2010): 29–37.

Niemi, Maria E., Mats Malqvist, Kim Bao Giang, Peter Allebeck, and Torkel Falkenberg. 2013. A narrative review of factors influencing detection and treatment of depression in Vietnam. *International Journal of Mental Health Systems* 7(15).

Ninh, Kim N. B. 2002. *A world transformed: The politics of culture in revolutionary Vietnam, 1945–1965.* Ann Arbor: University of Michigan Press.

Nonini, Donald. 2008. Is China becoming neoliberal? *Critique of Anthropology* 28(2): 145–176.

Nussbaum, Martha. 2001. *Upheavals of thought: The intelligence of emotions.* Cambridge: Cambridge University Press.

Obeyesekere, Gananath. 1990. *The work of culture: Symbolic transformation in psychoanalysis and anthropology.* Chicago: University of Chicago Press.

O'Gorman, Francis. 2015. *Worry: A literary and cultural history.* New York: Bloomsbury Academic.

Ong, Aihwa, and Li Zhang. 2008. Privatizing China: Powers of the self, socialism from afar. In *Privatizing China: Socialism from afar.* Li Zhang and Aihwa Ong, eds. Ithaca, NY: Cornell University Press. Pp. 1–20.

Osborne, Milton. 1980. The Indochinese refugees: Causes and effects. *International Affairs* 56(1): 37–53.

Ots, Thomas. 1990. The angry liver, the anxious heart, and the melancholy spleen. *Culture, Medicine, and Psychiatry* 14(1): 21–58.

Padilla, Mark B., Jennifer S. Hirsch, Miguel Munoz Laboy, Robert Sember, and Richard G. Parker, eds. 2008. *Love and globalization: Transformations of intimacy in the contemporary world.* Nashville, TN: Vanderbilt University Press.

Pandian, Anand. 2009. *Crooked stalks: cultivating virtue in South India.* Duke University Press.

Parish, Steven M. 1991. The sacred mind: Newar cultural representations of mental life and the production of consciousness. *Ethos* 19(3): 313–351.

————. 2008. *Subjectivity and suffering in American culture: Possible selves.* New York: Palgrave Macmillan.

————. 2014. Between persons: How concepts of the person make moral experience possible. *Ethos* 42(1): 31–50.

Pashigian, Melissa J. 2009. The womb, infertility, and the vicissitudes of kin-relatedness in Vietnam. *Journal of Vietnamese Studies* 4(2): 34–68.

————. 2012. Counting one's way to the global stage: Enumeration, accountability, and reproductive success in Vietnam. *Positions* 20(2): 529–558.

Patel, Vikram. 2014. Why mental health matters to global health. *Transcultural Psychiatry* 56(6): 777–789.

Patel, Vikram, Shekhar Saxena, Crick Lund, Graham Thornicroft, Florence Baingana, Paul Bolton, Dan Chisholm, et al. 2018. The Lancet Commission on Global Mental Health and Sustainable Development. *The Lancet* 392(10157): 1553–1598.

Penn, Sean, dir. 2007. *Into the wild*. 2007. Los Angeles: Paramount Vantage.

Peters, Erica J. 2012. Cuisine and social status among urban Vietnamese, 1888–1926. In *The reinvention of distinction: Modernity and the middle class in urban Vietnam*. Van Nguyen-Marshall, Lisa Welch Drummond, and Melanie Belanger, eds. Singapore: Asia Research Institute. Pp. 43–58.

Pettus, Ashley. 2003. *Between sacrifice and desire: National identity and the governing of femininity in Vietnam*. New York: Routledge.

Phan, Tuong, and Derrick Silove. 1997. The influence of culture on psychiatric assessment: The Vietnamese refugee. *Psychiatric Services* 48(1): 86–90.

———. 1999. An overview of indigenous descriptions of mental phenomena and the range of traditional healing practices amongst the Vietnamese. *Transcultural Psychiatry* 36(1): 79–94.

Phan, Tuong, Zachary Steel, and Derrick Silove. 2004. An ethnographically derived measure of anxiety, depression and somatization: The Phan Vietnamese Psychiatric Scale. *Transcultural Psychiatry* 41(2): 200–232.

Phinney, Harriet P. 2008a. Objects of affection: Vietnamese discourses on love and emancipation. *Positions* 16(2): 329–358.

———. 2008b. "Rice is essential but tiresome; you should get some noodles": *Doi moi* and the political economy of men's extramarital sexual relations and marital HIV risk in Hanoi, Vietnam. *American Journal of Public Health* 98(4): 650–660.

Povinelli, Elizabeth A. 2006. *The empire of love: Toward a theory of intimacy, genealogy, and carnality*. Durham, NC: Duke University Press.

Pritzker, Sonya E. 2016. New age with Chinese characteristics? Translating inner child emotion pedagogies in contemporary China. *Ethos* 44(2): 150–170.

———. 2020. Language, emotion, and the politics of vulnerability. *Annual Review of Anthropology* 49(1): 241–256.

Pritzker, Sonya E., and Whitney L. Duncan. 2019. Technologies of the social: Family constellation therapy and the remodeling of relational selfhood in China and Mexico. *Culture, Medicine, and Psychiatry* 43: 468–495.

Quinn, Naomi. 1987. Convergent evidence for a cultural model of marriage. In *Cultural models in language and thought*. Dorothy Holland and Naomi Quinn, eds. Cambridge: Cambridge University Press. Pp. 173–193.

Quinn, Naomi, and Dorothy Holland. 1987. Culture and cognition. In *Cultural models in language and thought*. Dorothy Holland and Naomi Quinn, eds. Cambridge: Cambridge University Press.

Quinn, Neil, Billy Bromage, and Michael Rowe. 2020. Collective citizenship: From citizenship and mental health to citizenship and solidarity. *Social Policy and Administration* 54(3): 361–374.

Rashid, Sabina Faiz. 2007. *Durbolota* (weakness), *chinta rog* (worry illness), and poverty: Explanations of white discharge among married adolescent women in a slum in Dhaka, Bangladesh. *Medical Anthropology Quarterly* 21(1): 108–132.

Rebhun, Linda A. 1999. *The heart is unknown country: Love in the changing economy of northeast Brazil*. Palo Alto, CA: Stanford University Press.

Redfield, Peter. 2005. Doctors, borders, and life in crisis. *Cultural Anthropology* 20(3): 328–361.

Richards, Analiese, and Daromir Rudnyckyj. 2009. Economies of affect. *Journal of the Royal Anthropological Institute* 15(1): 57–77.

Robbins, Joel. 2004. *Becoming sinners: Christianity and moral torment in a Papua New Guinea society*. Berkeley: University of California Press.

———. 2013. Beyond the suffering subject: toward an anthropology of the good. *Journal of the Royal Anthropological Institute* 19(3): 447–462.

Rofel, Lisa. 2007. *Desiring China: Experiments in neoliberalism, sexuality, and public culture*. Durham, NC: Duke University Press.

Roland, Douglas, and Daniel Jurafsky. 2002. Verb sense and verb subcategorization probabilities. In *The lexical basis of sentence processing: Formal, computational, and experimental issues*. Paola Merlo and Suzanne Stevenson, eds. Pp. 303–324.

Rosaldo, Michelle Z. 1983. The shame of headhunters and the autonomy of self. *Ethos* 11(3): 135–151.

Rose, Nikolas. 1992. Engineering the human soul: Analyzing psychological expertise. *Science in Context* 5(2): 351–369.

———. 1999. *Powers of freedom: Reframing political thought*. Cambridge: Cambridge University Press.

———. 2006. *The politics of life itself: Biomedicine, power, and subjectivity in the twenty-first century*. Princeton, NJ: Princeton University Press.

———. 2019. *Our psychiatric future*. Cambridge: Polity Press.

Rose, Nikolas, Nick Manning, Richard Bental, Kamaldeep Bhui, Rochelle Burgess, Sarah Carr, Flora Cornish, Delan Devakumar, Jennifer B. Dowd, Stefan Ecks, Alison Faulkner, Alex Ruck Keene, et al. 2020. The social underpinnings of mental distress in the time of COVID-19—time for urgent action. *Wellcome Open Research* 13(5): 166.

Rossi, Norma. 2017. The politics of anxiety and the rise of far-right parties in Europe. In *Politics of Anxiety*. Emmy Eklundh, Andreja Zevnik, and Emmanuel-Pierre Guittet, eds. London: Rowman & Littlefield International. Pp. 123–140.

Rudnyckyj, Daromir. 2011. Circulating tears and managing hearts: Governing through affect in an Indonesian steel factory. *Anthropological Theory* 11(1): 63–87.

Ryang, Sonia. 2006. *Love in modern Japan: Its estrangement from self, sex, and society*. London: Routledge.

Ryder, Andrew G., and Yulia E. Chentsova-Dutton. 2012. Depression in cultural context: "Chinese somatization," revisited. *Psychiatric Clinic of North America* 35(1): 15–36.

Rydstrøm, Helle. 2003a. *Embodying morality: Growing up in rural northern Vietnam*. Honolulu: University of Hawai'i Press.

———. 2003b. Encountering "hot" anger: Domestic violence in contemporary Vietnam. *Violence against Women* 9(6): 676–697.

———. 2006a. Masculinity and punishment: Men's upbringing of boys in rural Vietnam. *Childhood* 13(3): 329–348.

———. 2006b. Sexual desires and "social evils": Young women in rural Vietnam. *Gender, Place, and Culture* 13(3).

Salecl, Renata. 2004. *On anxiety*. London: Routledge.

———. 2020. *A passion for ignorance: What we choose not to know and why*. Princeton, NJ: Princeton University Press.

Schwartz, Barry. 2004. *The paradox of choice: Why more is less*. New York: Harper Perennial.

Schwenkel, Christina. 2012. Civilizing the city: Socialist ruins and urban renewal in Central Vietnam. *Positions* 20(2): 437–470.

———. 2013. Post/socialist affect: Ruination and reconstruction of the nation in urban Vietnam. *Cultural Anthropology* 28(2): 252–277.

Schwenkel, Christina, and Ann Marie Leshkowich. 2012. How is neoliberalism good to think Vietnam? How is Vietnam good to think neoliberalism? *Positions* 20(2): 379–401.

Seale-Feldman, Aidan. 2020. The work of disaster: Building back otherwise in post-earthquake Nepal. *Cultural Anthropology* 35(2): 237–263.

Searles, Edmund Q. 2000. "Why do you ask so many questions?": Dialogical anthropology and learning how not to ask in Canadian Inuit society. *Journal for the Anthropological Study of Human Movement* 11(1): 47–64.

Seigworth, Gregory J., and Melissa Gregg. 2010. An inventory of shimmers. In *The affect theory reader*. Melissa Gregg and Gregory J. Seigworth, eds. Durham, NC: Duke University Press. Pp. 1–25.

Shelley, Mary. 1818 (2003). *Frankenstein*. New York: Penguin Classics.

Shohet, Merav. 2013. Everyday sacrifice and language socialization in Vietnam: The power of a respect particle. *American Anthropologist* 115(2): 203–217.

———. 2017. Troubling love: Gender, class, and sideshadowing the "happy family" in Vietnam. *Ethos* 45(4): 555–576.

———. 2018. Two deaths and a funeral: Ritual inscriptions' affordances for mourning and moral personhood in Vietnam. *American Ethnologist* 45(1): 60–73.

———. 2021. *Silence and sacrifice: Family stories of care and the limits of love in Vietnam*. Oakland: University of California Press.

Shore, Bradd. 1996. *Culture in mind: Cognition, culture, and the problem of meaning*. Oxford: Oxford University Press.

Shweder, Richard A., and Edmund J. Bourne. 1984. Does the concept of person vary cross-culturally? In *Culture theory: Essays on mind, self, and emotion*. Richard A. Shweder and Robert A. Levine, eds. Cambridge: Cambridge University Press. Pp. 158–199.

Silberman, Steve. 2015. *Neurotribes: The legacy of autism and the future of neurodiversity*. New York: Penguin Random House.

Silva, Jennifer M. 2013. *Coming up short: Working-class adulthood in an age of uncertainty*. Oxford: Oxford University Press.

Singer, Judy. 1999. "Why can't you be normal for once in your life?" From a "problem with no name" to the emergence of a new category of difference. In *Disability discourse*. Mairian Corker and Sally French, eds. Philadelphia: Open University Press. Pp. 59–67.

Skidmore, Monique. 2003. Darker than midnight: Fear, vulnerability, and terror making in urban Burma (Myanmar). *American Ethnologist* 30(1): 5–21.

Skultans, Vieda. 1995. Neurasthenia and political resistance in Latvia. *Anthropology Today* 11(3): 14–18.

Small, Ivan V. 2018. *Currencies of imagination: Channeling money and chasing mobility in Vietnam*. Ithaca, NY: Cornell University Press.

Solomon, Andrew. 2001. *Noonday demon: An atlas of depression*. New York: Scribner.

Somers, Julian M., Elliott M. Goldner, and Paul Waraich. 2006. Prevalence and incidence studies of anxiety disorders: A systematic review of the literature. *The Canadian Journal of Psychiatry* 51(2): 100–113.

Soucy, Alexander. 2001. Romantic love and gender hegemony in Vietnam. In *Love, sex, and power: Women in Southeast Asia*. Susan Blackburn, ed. Clayton, Australia: Monash University Press. Pp. 31–41.

Stevenson, Lisa. 2014. *Life beside itself: Imagining care in the Canadian Arctic*. Oakland: University of California Press.

Stewart, Kathleen. 2007. *Ordinary affects*. Durham, NC: Duke University Press.

———. 2010. Worlding refrains. In *The affect theory reader*. Melissa Gregg and Gregory J. Seigworth, eds. Durham, NC: Duke University Press. Pp. 339–353.

Stone, Lawrence. 1977. *The family, sex and marriage in England, 1500–1800*. New York: Harper Colophon Books.

Stout, Noelle M. 2014. *After love: Queer intimacy and erotic economies in post-Soviet Cuba*. Durham, NC: Duke University Press.

Strauss, Claudia. 2006. The imaginary. *Anthropological Theory* 6(3): 322–334.

Sullivan, Harry Stack. 1948. The meaning of anxiety in psychiatry and in life. *Psychiatry* 11(1): 1–13.

Summerfield, Derek. 2008. How scientifically valid is the knowledge base of global mental health? *British Medical Journal* 336: 3509.

Szasz, Thomas S. 2001. The therapeutic state: The tyranny of pharmacracy. *The Independent Review* 5(4): 485–521.

Tai, Hue-Tam Ho. 1992. *Radicalism and the origins of the Vietnamese revolution*. Cambridge, MA: Harvard University Press.

———. 2001. Faces of remembering and forgetting. In *The country of memory: Remaking the past in Vietnam*. Hue-Tam Ho Tai, ed. Berkeley: University of California Press. Pp. 167–195.

Tan, Jonathan Y. 2016. A daughter's filiality, a courtesan's moral propriety, and a wife's conjugal love: Rethinking Confucian ethics for women in the Tale of Kiều. In *Religion and culture in dialogue*. J. Talivaldis Ozolins, ed. New York: Springer. P. 15.

Tang, Xiaobing. 2000. *Chinese modern: The heroic and the quotidian*. Durham, NC: Duke University Press.

Taylor, Charles. 1989. *Sources of the self: The making of the modern identity*. Cambridge, MA: Harvard University Press.

Taylor, Keith W. 1983. *The birth of Vietnam*. Berkeley: University of California Press.

Taylor, Nora. 2012. Exhibiting middle classless: The social status of artists in Hanoi. In *The reinvention of distinction: Modernity and the middle class in urban Vietnam*. Van Nguyen-Marshall, Lisa Welch Drummond, and Melanie Belanger, eds. Singapore: Asia Research Institute. Pp. 115–128.

Taylor, Philip. 2001. *Fragments of the present: Searching for modernity in Vietnam's south*. Honolulu: University of Hawai'i Press.

Throop, C. Jason. 2003. Articulating experience. *Anthropological Theory* 3(2): 219–241.

———. 2010a. Latitudes of loss: On the vicissitudes of empathy. *American Ethnologist* 37(4): 771–781.

———. 2010b. *Suffering and sentiment: Exploring the vicissitudes of experience and pain in Yap*. Berkeley: University of California Press.

———. 2012. Moral sentiments. In *A companion to moral anthropology*. Didier Fassin, ed. Hoboken, NJ: Wiley.

———. 2014. Moral moods. *Ethos* 42: 65–83.

Thuý Hạnh. December 7, 2015. Gần 14 triệu người Việt bị rối loạn tâm thần [Almost 14 million Vietnamese have mental illness]. *Vietnamnet*. Retrieved from http://vietnamnet.vn.

Tran, Allen L. 2015. Rich sentiments and the cultural politics of emotion in postreform Ho Chi Minh City, Vietnam. *American Anthropologist* 117(3): 480–492.

———. 2017. Neurasthenia, generalized anxiety disorder, and the medicalization of worry in a Vietnamese psychiatric hospital. *Medical Anthropology Quarterly* 31: 198–217.

———. 2018. The anxiety of romantic love in Ho Chi Minh City, Vietnam. *Journal of the Royal Anthropological Institute* 24: 512–531.

Tran, Allen L., Trần Đan Tâm, Hà Thúc Dũng, and Nguyễn Cúc Trâm. 2020. Drug adherence, medical pluralism, and psychopharmaceutical selfhood in postreform Vietnam. *Transcultural Psychiatry* 57(1): 81–93.

Trinh, Binh. 2022. The moral middle-class in market socialism: An investigation into the personhood of women working in NGOs in Vietnam. *Asian Journal of Social Science* 50(2): 104–111.

Truitt, Allison. 2008. On the back of a motorbike: Middle-class mobility in Ho Chi Minh City, Vietnam. *American Ethnologist* 35(1): 3–19.

Trương Huyền Chi. 2009. A home divided: Work, body, and emotion in the post *đổi mới*-family. In *Reconfiguring families in contemporary Vietnam*. Danielle Belanger and Magali Barbieri, eds. Palo Alto, CA: Stanford University Press. Pp. 298–328.

Turley, William S. 1993. Introduction. In *Reinventing Vietnamese socialism: Đổi mới in comparative perspective*. William S. Turley and Mark Seldon, eds. Boulder, CO: Westview Press. Pp. 1–15.

Turner, R. Jay, B. Gail Frankel, and Deborah M. Levin. 1983. Social support: Conceptualization, measurement, and implications for mental health. *Research in Community & Mental Health* 3: 67–111.

Urciuoli, Bonnie. 2008. Skills and selves in the new workplace. *American Ethnologist* 35(2): 211–228.

Vann, Elizabeth. 2012. Consumption and middle-class subjectivity in Vietnam. In *The reinvention of distinction: Modernity and the middle class in urban Vietnam*. Van Nguyen-Marshall, Lisa Welch Drummond, and Melanie Belanger, eds. Singapore: Asia Research Institute. Pp. 157–170.

Viện Ngôn ngữ học [Institute of Linguistics]. 2002. *Từ điển Tiếng Việt Phổ thông* [Popular Vietnamese Dictionary]. Hanoi: NXB Từ điển Bách khoa [Polytechnic Dictionary Press].

Virno, Paolo. 2004. *A grammar of the multitude: For an analysis of contemporary forms of life*. Cambridge, MA: MIT Press.

Vu, Thanh Thi. 2020. Love, affection, and intimacy in marriage of young people in Vietnam. *Asian Studies Review* 45(1): 100–116.

Wagner, Renate, Vijaya Manicavasagar, Derrick Silove, Claire Marnane, and Viet Thang Tran. 2006. Characteristics of Vietnamese patients attending an anxiety clinic in Australia and perceptions of the wider Vietnamese community about anxiety. *Transcultural Psychiatry* 43(2): 259–274.

Wahlberg, Ayo, and Nikolas Rose. 2015. The governmentalization of living: Calculating global health. *Economy and Society* 44(1): 60–90.

Weber, Samuel. 1991. *Return to Freud: Jacques Lacan's dislocation of psychoanalysis*. Michael Levine, trans. Cambridge: Cambridge University Press.

Weiss, Mitchell. 1997. Explanatory Model Interview Catalogue (EMIC): Framework for comparative study of illness. *Transcultural Psychiatry* 34(2): 235–263.

WHO World Mental Health Survey Consortium. 2004. Prevalence, severity, and unmet need for treatment of mental disorders in the World Health Organization world mental health surveys. *JAMA* 291(21): 2581–2590.

Wicks, Robert. 2009. French existentialism. In *A companion to phenomenology and existentialism*. Hubert L. Dreyfuss and Mark A. Wrathall, eds. Oxford: Blackwell. Pp. 209–227.

Wilce, James M. 2003. *Eloquence in trouble: The poetics and politics of complaint in rural Bangladesh*. Oxford: Oxford University Press.

Wilce, James M., and Janina Fenigsen. 2016. Emotion pedagogies: What are they, and why do they matter? *Ethos* 44 (2): 81–95.

Willen, Sarah S. 2007. Toward a critical phenomenology of "illegality": State power, criminalization, and objectivity among undocumented migrant workers in Tel Aviv, Israel. *International Migration* 45(3): 8–48.

———. 2019. *Fighting for dignity: Migrant lives at Israel's margin*. Philadelphia: University of Pennsylvania Press.

Williams, Alex. June 10, 2017. Prozac Nation is now the United States of Xanax. *The New York Times*. https://www.nytimes.com/2017/06/10/style/anxiety-is-the-new-depression-xanax.html (retrieved September 20, 2019).

Williams, Lindy, and Michael Guest. 2005. Attitudes towards marriage among the urban middle-class in Vietnam, Thailand, and the Philippines. *Journal of Comparative Family Studies* 36.

Williams, Raymond. 1977. *Marxism and literature*. Oxford: Oxford University Press.

Wilson, Ara. 2004. *Intimate economies of Bangkok: Tomboys, tycoons, and Avon ladies in the global city*. Berkeley: University of California Press.

World Bank & Ministry of Planning and Investment of Vietnam. 2016. *Vietnam 2035: Toward prosperity, creativity, equity, and democracy*. Washington, DC: World Bank. https://openknowledge.worldbank.org/handle/10986/23724.

World Health Organization. 2014. *Social determinants of mental health*. Geneva: World Health Organization.

———. 2021. *Guidance on community mental health services: Promoting person-centered and rights-based approaches*. Geneva: World Health Organization.

Yan, Yunxiang. 2003. *Private life under socialism: Love, intimacy, and family change in a Chinese village, 1949–1999*. Palo Alto, CA: Stanford University Press.

———. 2010. The Chinese path to individualization. *British Journal of Sociology* 61(3): 489–512.

———. 2011. The changing moral landscape. In *Deep China: The moral life of the person*. Arthur Kleinman, Yunxiang Yan, Jing Jun, Sing Lee, and Everett Zhang, eds. Berkeley: University of California Press. Pp. 36–77.

Yang, Jie. 2013. "Fake happiness": Counseling, potentiality, and psychopolitics in China. *Ethos* 41(3): 292–312.

———. 2014. "The happiness of the marginalized": Affect, counseling, and self-reflexivity in China. In *The political economy of affect and emotion in East Asia*. Jie Yang, ed. New York: Routledge. Pp. 45–62.

———. 2017. *Mental health in China: Change, tradition, and therapeutic governance.* Medford, MA: Polity Press.

Yarris, Kristin E. 2011. The pain of "thinking too much": Dolor de cerebro and the embodiment of social hardship among Nicaraguan women. *Ethos* 39(2): 226–248.

Yates-Doerr, Emily. 2015. *The weight of obesity: Hunger and global health in postwar Guatemala.* Oakland: University of California Press.

Zhang, Li. 2012. Afterword: Flexible postsocialist assemblages from the margin. *Positions* 20(2): 659–667.

———. 2014. Bentuhua: Psychotherapy in postsocialist China. *Culture, Medicine, and Psychiatry* 38: 283–305.

———. 2017. The rise of therapeutic governing in postsocialist China. *Medical Anthropology* 36(1): 6–18.

———. 2018. Cultivating the therapeutic self in China. *Medical Anthropology* 37(1): 45–58.

———. 2020. *Anxious China: Inner revolution and politics of psychotherapy.* Oakland: University of California Press.

Zhou, Xiaolu, Jessica Dere, Xiongzhao Zhu, Shuqiao Yao, Yulia Chentsova-Dutton, and Andrew Ryder. 2011. Anxiety symptom presentations in Han Chinese and Euro-Canadian outpatients: Is distress always somatized in China? *Journal of Affective Disorders* 135: 111–114.

Zigon, Jarrett. 2007. Moral breakdown and the ethical demand: A theoretical framework for an anthropology of moralities. *Anthropological Theory* 7 (2): 131–150.

———. 2010. Moral and ethical assemblages. *Anthropological Theory* 10 (1–2): 3–15.

———. 2013. On love: Remaking moral subjectivity in postrehabilitation Russia. *American Ethnologist* 40: 201–215.

———. 2019. *A war on people: Drug user politics and a new ethics of community.* Oakland: University of California Press.

———. 2021. How is it between us? Relational ethics and transcendence. *Journal of the Royal Anthropological Institute* 27: 384–401.

Žižek, Slavoj. 1989. *The sublime object of ideology.* Brooklyn, NY: Verso.

INDEX

Founded in 1893,
UNIVERSITY OF CALIFORNIA PRESS
publishes bold, progressive books and journals
on topics in the arts, humanities, social sciences,
and natural sciences—with a focus on social
justice issues—that inspire thought and action
among readers worldwide.

The UC PRESS FOUNDATION
raises funds to uphold the press's vital role
as an independent, nonprofit publisher, and
receives philanthropic support from a wide
range of individuals and institutions—and from
committed readers like you. To learn more, visit
ucpress.edu/supportus.